OXFORD MEDICAL PUBLICATIONS

Medical Emergencies in Dentistry

Published and forthcoming titles in the Emergencies in... series:

Head, Neck and Dental Emergencies
Edited by Mike Perry

Emergencies in Anaesthesia
Edited by Keith Allman, Andrew McIndoe, and Iain H. Wilson

Emergencies in Cardiology
Saul G. Myerson, Robin P. Choudhury, and Andrew Mitchell

Emergencies in Obstetrics and Gynaecology
Edited by S. Arulkumaran

Medical Emergencies in Dentistry
Nigel D. Robb and Jason Leitch

Emergencies in Palliative and Supportive Care
Edited by David Currow and Katherine Clark

Medical Emergencies in Dentistry

Nigel D. Robb

Senior Lecturer in Sedation in Relation to Dentistry,
Glasgow Dental Hospital and School,
Glasgow, UK

Jason Leitch

Clinical Lecturer in Oral Surgery,
Glasgow Dental Hospital and School,
Glasgow, UK and
Health Foundation Fellow, Institute for Healthcare
Improvement, Cambridge, MA 02138, USA

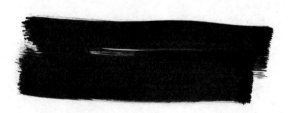

OXFORD
UNIVERSITY PRESS

OXFORD
UNIVERSITY PRESS

Great Clarendon Street, Oxford OX2 6DP

Oxford University Press is a department of the University of Oxford.
It furthers the University's objective of excellence in research, scholarship,
and education by publishing worldwide in

Oxford New York

Auckland Cape Town Dar es Salaam Hong Kong Karachi
Kuala Lumpur Madrid Melbourne Mexico City Nairobi
New Delhi Shanghai Taipei Toronto

With offices in

Argentina Austria Brazil Chile Czech Republic France Greece
Guatemala Hungary Italy Japan Poland Portugal Singapore
South Korea Switzerland Thailand Turkey Ukraine Vietnam

Oxford is a registered trade mark of Oxford University Press
in the UK and in certain other countries

Published in the United States
by Oxford University Press Inc., New York

British Library Cataloguing in Publication Data
Data available

Library of Congress Cataloging in Publication Data
Data available

Typeset by Newgen Imaging Systems (P) Ltd., Chennai, India
Printed in Italy
on acid-free paper by LegoPrint S.p.A

ISBN 0-19-852931-7 (flexicover:alk.paper)   978-0-19-852931-6 (flexicover:alk.paper)

10 9 8 7 6 5 4 3 2 1

Preface

Emergencies by their nature require an immediate response. They also occur infrequently. Consequently both knowledge and practical skills for managing medical emergencies in a dental setting must be available for immediate implementation by all dental care personnel. Many dentists have anxieties about providing care for patients with medical problems solely due to lack of confidence in their own emergency management skills. The UK General Dental Council (GDC) core ethical guidance 'Standards for Dental Professionals' states that all members of the dental team must train and prepare together so that all can fulfil their role in such an emergency. With the support of the GDC, guidance from the UK Resuscitation Council has given the dental profession nationally agreed core drugs, equipment, and training standards. Thus recognition and management of medical emergencies should form part of continued professional development for all dental care professionals throughout their practising careers.

Competence comes both from knowledge and skills and in this book Drs Robb and Leitch have prepared a concise factual base upon which practical training can be built. Those of us involved in training undergraduates and postgraduates in the management of medical emergencies realise that key information needs to be clearly stated. In this handbook the reader will find short and memorable lists of features of medical emergencies to help with diagnosis and the management appropriate in a dental primary care setting. This book should be part of every dentist and dental student's collection as it is a clear and practical guide to one of the most important aspects of patient care.

Dr Alexander J. Crighton
BDS, MB ChB(Edin), FDS RCPS, FDS (OM) RCSEd,
Consultant in Oral Medicine
Honorary Senior Lecturer in Medicine
in Relation to Dentistry
Glasgow Dental Hospital and School.

Acknowledgements

The authors would like to acknowledge the help of Mr Rod Miller, clinical photographer at Glasgow Dental Hospital and School for his help in the production of the illustrations in this text. They would also like to thank the Resuscitation Council for their permission to reproduce the ALS algorithm as Fig. 10.5 and Laerdal UK for their permission to reproduce the 'chain of survival' as Fig. 10.1.

NDR, JL
2006

Contents

Detailed Contents

Introduction

The management of medical emergencies is an area that frequently arouses feelings of panic amongst members of the dental profession. Such feelings are often the result of fear of the unknown. Fortunately, as is described in Chapter 2, the incidence of medical emergencies in the dental setting is extremely small. However, this brings its own problems, as the chances of anyone in the dental team having encountered any of the emergencies is likewise small. There is therefore little opportunity to draw on the experience of others to help with the management of medical problems.

The requirement of effective preparation is thus increased because of the rarity of such events. This is emphasized by the General Dental Council, who stated in the 2001 version of *Maintaining Standards*[1] that the whole of the dental team should practice the management of simulated medical emergencies, against the clock, on a regular basis. Although this document has now been superseded by *Standards for Dental Professionals*[2], the duty of care which a dentist and their team accept when treating a patient should include not only the management of the complications of that treatment but also the management of medical incidents within the dental environment. The recent increased availability of automated external defibrillators in some retail shops and railway stations means that there is a greater expectation on the dental profession to provide trained help.

This text aims to provide an easy-to-use guide that will take the reader through the main diagnostic features and principles of management of the medical incidents that are seen most commonly within the practice of dentistry.

The main intention of this book is to ensure that the basics of management of medical emergencies are carried out to a high standard.

1 *Maintaining standards* (2001) General Dental Council, London.
2 *Standards for dental professionals* (2005) General Dental Council, London.

Contents of the book

Chapter 2 covers risk assessment and preparation. It is often incorrectly assumed that medical emergencies cannot be predicted or prevented. Many medical emergencies can be anticipated and, with the correct management, be prevented. The term 'risk assessment' is gaining much popularity in management circles, and whilst this text will not give an in-depth account of the process it will indicate a strategy that can be adopted to minimize the potential problems that might be encountered in the dental environment.

The medical emergencies are covered in chapters relating to the systems that are affected. The circulatory emergencies relate to emergencies that affect the flow of blood as a result of alteration to the way the blood is able to flow through blood vessels, whilst the cardiovascular system emergencies relate to alterations in the efficacy of the heart in pumping blood. Events affecting the central nervous system and respiratory tract, as well as those arising from hormonal imbalance, are described.

Some types of medical emergency are difficult to classify. Anaphylaxis, for example, affects both the circulatory system (by causing widespread vasodilation and fall in blood pressure) and the respiratory system (by causing severe bronchospasm and occlusion of the airway). In such cases, the description will be given in one chapter and cross-referenced to other potentially appropriate chapters.

Basic life support is accorded a chapter in its own right, although this is a technique for the management of cardiac arrest. The correct performance of basic life support is vital to the successful outcome of cardiac arrest, as well as providing principles that can be applied to all medical emergency management situations. Thus, the authors felt it best to deal with this issue in a separate chapter.

Immediate and advanced life support are only required in specific areas of dental practice. The arrival of a paramedic ambulance in response to an emergency call will be the time at which advanced life support commences. The chapter on immediate and advanced life support is included for information so that the dental team will understand the process that has been initiated by the emergency call. The description of immediate and advanced life support gives the context for the management that is undertaken in the dental environment.

What emergency drugs should be kept in dental practices?

There have been many recommendations published over the years as to what might be considered an appropriate level of drugs and equipment to keep in a dental practice. The most recent report emanated from Scotland[3] and looked to provide a simplified list of five drugs. The authors would commend this approach. It is anticipated that many readers may go through their entire practising lives without seeing some (or perhaps most of the conditions) described in this text. It is thus unreasonable to expect dental surgeons to remember long and complicated drug regimes that they are unlikely to ever use. The incidence of medical emergencies in dental practice and the drugs that have actually been used to manage them are reviewed in Chapter 2.

The authors also commend that the emergency drugs should be able to be administered by routes other than intravenously. The majority of dental surgeons do not practice gaining intravenous access regularly. Expecting them to do so in less than ideal circumstances is unreasonable.

It is not required that dental surgeons either have or know how to interpret electrocardiograms (ECG). Thus, none of the drugs that are recommended should either need an ECG diagnosis or should their use demand continual monitoring with an ECG because of potential side-effects.

The emergency drugs that are recommended are shown in Table 1.1 along with the routes by which they can be administered. This list is a minimum for all dental practices. It does not preclude other drugs being added. For example, hypostop (a glucose preparation that is absorbed across the oral mucosa) could be additional to glucagon. This list also does not cover practices where conscious sedation is used. In that situation, if there are antagonist drugs for the sedative agents they must be available in the practice. Table 1.2 lists these drugs.

It is also the authors' belief that, as a fundamental principle, the dental surgeon in the practice should be able to use the drugs that are kept in that practice. It is pointless keeping a selection of drugs in the hope that someone who might be able to use them will arrive to help.

3 Wray D (Chairman, National Dental Advisory Committee) (1999) *Emergency dental drugs: report of an expert working party*. Scottish Office, Department of Health, Edinburgh.

Table 1.1 Recommended emergency drug list for all dental practices

Drug	Routes of administration	Principal indication
Oxygen	Inhalation	All medical emergencies except hyperventilation
Adrenaline 1:1000	Intramuscular	Anaphylaxis
Salbutamol	Inhalation	Acute asthma
Glyceryl trinitrate	Sublingual	Angina
Glucagon	Intramuscular	Hypoglycaemia

Table 1.2 Additional drugs for practices providing conscious sedation

Sedation technique	Drugs to be available	Route of administration	Indication
Relative analgesia	No extra drugs required		
Intravenous benzodiazepine	Flumazenil	Intravenous	Oversedation
Oral benzodiazepine	Flumazenil	Intravenous	Oversedation
Multiple-agent intravenous sedation including opioids	Naloxone	Intravenous	Oversedation
Intravenous propofol	ALS drugs	Intravenous	See Chapter 10

What equipment should be stocked for management of medical emergencies?

The equipment that should be kept for the management of medical emergencies is given in Table 1.3. Again, the principle that has been adopted is that nothing that it would not be reasonable to use in dental practice has been included.

It is possible to obtain the emergency drugs listed in Table 1.1 in pre-loaded syringes. This has the advantage of saving the time and effort that is involved in drawing drugs up for emergency use. The disadvantage of this is that the preloaded syringes are more expensive than the combined cost of the same drug in ampule form and the equipment to then administer the drug. Drugs purchased in preloaded syringes also tend to have a shorter shelf life. The General Dental Council and Resuscitation Council advise that preloaded syringes are used. When the emergency drugs pass their expiry date they can be used for training and practise in drawing up drugs should the dental team feel that this would be appropriate.

The maintenance of the emergency drugs box must form part of the routine of the dental practice.

The other equipment that is required is designed to enable the airway to be cleared and maintained and the patient ventilated with exhaled air respiration. The equipment is simple to use and maintain.

It is important to have portable, independently powered suction as, although the dental aspirator will provide effective suction to clear the airway, it cannot be guaranteed that the victim of a collapse will be within range of the aspirator.

A pocket mask is preferred to a self-inflating bag, as it is easier to use for a single operator effectively; a properly used pocket mask is far better than a poorly used self-inflating bag.

Table 1.3 Equipment required for use in dental emergencies for all dental settings

Equipment	Notes
Portable, independently powered suction	
Yaunkauer suckers and suction catheters	Adult and paediatric sizes
Oral pharyngeal airways	Sizes 1, 2, 3, and 4
Pocket mask with oxygen inlet	For example, Laerdal mask
	Portex Safe Response
Portable oxygen with flow meter	Needs associated tubing and mask
1ml syringes	If preloaded syringes not used
Sterile disposable needles	21g × 1.75" (green)
	23g × 1.5" (blue)

Risk assessment

Introduction

Prior preparation prevents a poor performance. Prevention is better than cure. These are two sayings that have been applied to a number of areas of clinical practice and life in general. They are pertinent to the area of management of medical incidents in the dental environment. It would, however, be of benefit to all concerned if the medical incident could be prevented. Adequate preparation of the patient, coupled with an anticipation of when problems might arise will reduce the likelihood of medical incidents occurring. Still, it will not be possible to prevent all medical incidents. Such incidents are stressful for the patient and the dental team. However, proper preparation of the dental team will improve the team's performance when called upon to manage those medical incidents that cannot be prevented and to ensure that the patient has the best chance of survival and return to health. In turn, this will prevent feelings of guilt in members of the dental team, who otherwise might feel that they could have done better.

This chapter will consider the preparation of the patient to receive dental treatment and the preparation of the team to deal with medical incidents.

Incidence of medical emergencies in the practice of dentistry

It is important to put the risk of encountering a medical emergency in context. The incidence of medical emergencies during the practice of dentistry is low (as will be seen later). The majority of dental personnel will have little experience of managing medical emergencies. Part of the risk assessment must, therefore, be the preparation of the dental team to deal with medical emergencies. The premise in this text is that the dental practice will be equipped as outlined in Chapter 1. Training to use the recommended drugs and equipment is an integral part of the risk assessment process.

There has been little published research on the incidence of medical emergencies in the dental setting. The figures quoted here are from a series of papers published in 1999[1,2,3]. The study from which these figures are taken did not ask for details of the incidence of faints or reactions to intravascular injection of epinephrine containing local anaesthetic solutions. These events are thought to occur relatively frequently in practice and to be well managed by the dental team.

Seventy percent of the practitioners in this study reported having had at least one medical incident during a 10-year period in dental practice. Table 2.1 shows the number of emergency events reported in this study as well as the calculation of how many such events a dentist could expect to see in a practicing lifetime of 40 years. (These events were recorded for those who were not involved in the provision of general anaesthesia or conscious sedation.) Using the number of reported incidents (2101) and the total number of years' dental practice (8849) it can be calculated that there will be one event for every 4.2 years of practice.

In a practicing lifetime of approximately 40 years, a dentist can thus expect to see about 10 medical incidents. This is not a sufficient number to allow the dental team to maintain a level of competence in the management of such incidents without additional training—hence the need for continuing education in this area.

Types of event

The types of event that were found to occur were:
- Fits and seizures (about 33% of reports)
- Swallowed foreign bodies (about 16%)
- Angina pectoris (about 10%)
- Diabetic events (also about 10%).

1 Atherton GJ, McCaul JA, Williams SA (1999) Medical emergencies in general dental practice in Great Britain. Part 1: their prevalence over a 10-year period. *Brit Dent J* **186**:72–79.

2 Atherton GJ, McCaul JA, Williams SA (1999) Medical emergencies in general dental practice in Great Britain. Part 2: drugs and equipment possessed by GDPs and used in the management of emergencies. *Brit Dent J* **186**:125–130.

3 Atherton GJ, McCaul JA, Williams SA (1999) Medical emergencies in general dental practice in Great Britain. Part 3: perceptions of training and competence of GDPs in their management. *Brit Dent J* **186**:234–237.

The majority of the events are not potentially fatal, and with appropriate simple management the patient should make a complete recovery. It is also true that mismanagement can turn a minor event into a serious incident. It is thus important that the management is kept simple and yet effective. Simple so that there is less chance of inadvertently aggravating the situation, yet effective in order to manage the condition appropriately.

Table 2.1 Medical emergencies reported over a 10-year period and projected number expected during a 40-year working life in dental practice (after Atherton et al. 1999[1])

Event	Number reported	Number projected in 40-year dental practice career
Fits/seizures	699	3.16
Swallowed object	369	1.67
Asthma	286	1.29
Angina pectoris	237	1.07
Diabetic events	227	1.02
Drug reactions	180	0.81
Cardiac arrest	37	0.17
Myocardial infarction	25	0.11
Cerebrovascular accident	18	0.08
Inhaled object	13	0.06
Miscellaneous others	49	0.22

When do events occur?

The medical emergencies were most likely to occur during treatment (36.7%). The next most likely time was immediately following the administration of local anaesthesia (23.1%). There were more emergencies prior to treatment (23.1%) than after treatment (16.4%). Only a very small number (about 2%) occurred after the patient had returned home.

Stress is frequently an aggravating factor. Patients are likely to feel stressed during treatment, and this may account for the majority of medical incidents occurring during treatment. It is also well known that the anticipation of events is a cause of stress. This would account for the fact that more emergencies occur before rather than after treatment.

Who is affected?

The majority of the medical emergencies affected dental patients, with only about 2.5% affecting people who were not undergoing treatment. The 2.5% who were not having dental treatment included relatives accompanying patients, passers by whose assistance had been sought from the dental surgery, and also dental personnel. One incentive for a dental team well trained in the management of medical incidents is that this will ensure that any member of the team who suffers an unfortunate event is well looked after by his or her colleagues. It is encouraging that dental personnel are unlikely to be seriously affected at work.

What happens to the patients?

The data on the outcome of the medical emergencies was not reported in about a quarter of cases: despite this, it would appear that less than a quarter (23%) of medical emergencies in the dental environment result in referral to hospital. The most common reason for referral to hospital was for radiographic investigation of swallowed foreign bodies (36.9% of hospital referrals). Thus, only 16.8% of those who suffer a medical incident in the dental environment require treatment in hospital. (A radiographic examination to establish where a swallowed object is located is not counted as medical *treatment* but an *investigation*.)

What treatment is provided in the dental environment?

The most commonly treated medical emergency was a diabetic event, in which glucose was administered. The other 'commonly used' drugs were glyceryl trinitrate for angina pectoris and inhalers for the treatment of asthma. The only drugs that were administered by the dental team in the cumulative total of almost 9000 years of practice were:

- Oxygen
- Epinephrine
- Glyceryl trinitrate
- Salbutamol
- Chlorpheniramine
- Dextrose
- Hydrocortisone
- Midazolam.

The list of drugs which should be held in dental practices for the management of medical emergencies has been the subject of much debate. In 1990, the 'Poswillo' report[4] was published. This report recommended a list of 16 emergency drugs and an additional two solutions for infusion. The list given in Chapter 1 (see p. 7) was published in Scotland in 1999[5]. It contains five drugs, all of which were used by those who completed questionnaires in the studies we have quoted. The only additions to that list which could be considered, in the light of the evidence available, would be an oral sugar preparation and an anticonvulsant. The holding of a large number of drugs to manage medical incidents within the dental setting cannot be justified. It is the authors' opinion that the list as published in 1999[5] is perfectly adequate for dental settings.

How many patients have died?

In the almost 9000 years of practice, there were 20 deaths reported of which four affected passers by. In these cases, which all occurred in Scotland, three patients suffered a cardiac arrest and one a massive cerebrovascular accident near the dental surgery. In each case, staff from the

4 Poswillo DE (Chairman, Standing Dental Advisory Committee) (1990) *General anaesthesia, sedation and resuscitation in dentistry: report of an expert working party.* London, HMSO.

5 Wray D (Chairman, National Dental Advisory Committee) (1999) *Emergency dental drugs: report of an expert working party.* Scottish Office, Department of Health, Edinburgh.

dental practice offered assistance prior to the arrival of the emergency services. The incidence of death associated with the practice of dentistry in the UK is, thus, 16 in 8849 years or one every 553 years. Assuming that a career in dental practice lasts 40 years, there is a 1 in 14 chance of seeing a patient death.

Although these events are infrequent, prevention is still better than cure. Wherever possible, steps to prevent medical incidents should be taken. The first of these is to ensure that the patient is prepared.

Preparation of the patient

Medical emergencies in dentistry are rarely totally unpredictable. Many patients (or indeed dental personnel) have significant medical histories or signs that would indicate they are at risk of being the victim of a medical incident. Risk management involves the assessment of the patient for risk factors for medical emergencies.

Never treat a stranger! The old axiom is as valid in the twenty-first century as ever in the past. The advances in modern medicine and surgery result in outpatients surviving medical conditions that would have been fatal for their parents and grandparents. Modern pharmacology masks underlying signs of disease making patients appear fitter than they actually are. Many patients have the capacity to change from apparently fit to almost moribund in a short period (see section on hypoglycaemia, pp. 60–61). Hence the need for full assessment.

Knowing your patient involves obtaining information about their medical and dental history as well as providing a physical assessment.

Patient's medical history

The medical history is the basis of patient evaluation. It is both a moral and a General Dental Council requirement that patients who are to receive dental treatment should have a thorough medical history recorded. The normal way of obtaining a medical history is to use a written, patient-completed medical history questionnaire (Fig. 2.1 opposite).

The completed questionnaire provides the dentist with valuable information about the patient's physical status. In addition, it may also provide information about the patient's psychological status. The answers obtained from the questionnaire must be supplemented by the appropriate clinical history taking. Frequently, patients will be unaware of the names of all the medication they are taking. Drug interactions are a common cause of problems in dentistry (see Chapter 7). All patients must provide details of their medication prior to the start of treatment.

The past medical history, particularly the presence of chronic disease, provides a guide as to possible causes of collapse in the dental environment.

The medical history questionnaire shown in Fig. 2.1 has 16 questions. Positive answers to any questions are a prompt for further questioning. It is also important that negative answers are confirmed. The majority of patients do not intentionally lie to the dentist, but they may inadvertently over look something in their history or fail to see the importance of a piece of information. Often, this may be the taking of herbal remedies or over-the-counter medication. Many patients do not feel that these are as important as medicines that are prescribed by a doctor.

While it is beyond the scope of this text to consider all of the possible conditions that may affect the patient, some examples of the assistance that can be obtained from a medical history are given.

<u>Conscious Sedation Treatment Record</u>

| Patient label | ASSESSMENT DATE |
| | PROPOSED PROCEDURE |

GLASGOW
DENTAL
HOSPITAL
& SCHOOL

Date _____ History taker (Print) _____	Yes	No
1. Do you have a history of heart murmur, heart disease, or cardiac surgery?		
2. Do you suffer from asthma or other form of chest disease?		
3. Have you ever had a general anaesthetic or sedation before?		
4. Have you had any problems with any previous general anaesthetic or sedation?		
5. Is there any family history of problems with general anaesthetics or sedation?		
6. Are you taking any prescribed medicines (tablets, creams, ointments or inhalers)?		
7. Are you allergic to any medicines, foods or other substances?		
8. Have you suffered from epilepsy or regular faints?		
9. Do you suffer from epilepsy or regular faints?		
10. Have you ever suffered from rheumatic fever?		
11. Do you suffer from diabetes?		
12. Have you had steroid medication within the last two years?		
13. Have you had episodes of spontaneous bleeding or prolonged bleeding after surgery?		
14. Have you ever been in hospital?		
15 Are you currently attending a doctor, hospital or other specialist?		
16. Is there any matter not covered above that you feel we should know?		
Further Details		

I believe the above information to be correct

Signature _____ Relationship to patient _____

Fig. 2.1

Question 1

A patient with a history of stress- or exercise-induced angina will be susceptible to the stress of dental treatment. Such individuals will also potentially require a reduction in the maximum amount of epinephrine-containing local anaesthetic administered. Keeping the stress of dental treatment to a minimum and sensible dose limitation in local anaesthetic solution will thus decrease the likelihood of an angina attack occurring during dental treatment.

A patient whose angina has an atypical presentation, occurring spontaneously or where the severity of symptoms is at great risk, should not receive elective treatment until the medical condition has been treated.

A patient who has a history of myocardial infarction (MI) will be at extra risk of repeat infarction in the first three months post MI.

Question 2

Asthma is a very common condition. Acute exacerbations can be induced by stress. Dentally anxious patients who also have asthma may have stress-induced attacks in the dental setting. The best guides to the severity of a patient's asthma are the frequency of attacks and the frequency of the use of inhalers. A history of asthma can also be an indication of an increased likelihood of other atopic symptoms.

Questions 3, 4, and 5

In addition to providing information regarding possible adverse drug reactions, these questions will give an indication of the way that the patient has received dental treatment previously. Patients who have a long history of receiving treatment under general anaesthesia or sedation are likely to be anxious about dental treatment.

Question 6

The patient's drug history is important for a number of reasons:

- Firstly, direct therapeutic effects of the drug may influence the dental treatment of the patient. For example, patients taking warfarin are prone to postoperative bleeding.
- Secondly, the side-effects of a drug may affect patients' responses to treatment. For example, many agents used to treat hypertension can cause postural hypotension which can increase the chance of a faint once treatment is completed and the patient is moved from the supine to the upright position.
- Thirdly, there is the possibility of drug interactions. This subject is covered in Chapter 7.
- Fourthly, the patient's drug history is an indication of the medical history. Patients taking antihypertensive therapies will have underlying hypertension. Hypertension is a predisposing factor for cerebrovascular accidents (strokes)—see Chapter 8.

Question 7

Allergies to therapeutic agents will limit what can be prescribed. Positive answers should be followed up as many patients indicate that they are allergic to an agent when they have experienced symptoms that are normal drug side-effects. For example, gastrointestinal upset on antimicrobials such as erythromycin.

Potential allergens in the dental surgery also include latex and sticking plasters that might be used after intravenous sedation.

Question 8

A past history of hepatitis may indicate an exposure to one of the hepatitis viruses. Whilst this is an issue in terms of infection control, it will not affect dental treatment. A patient who is jaundiced or has impaired hepatic function may be unable to metabolize drugs as efficiently as patients with normal hepatic function. Patients with hepatic impairment may have impaired blood clotting leading to increased postoperative haemorrhage.

Question 9

A positive answer to a history of fits may indicate the presence of epilepsy. Stress is an inducing factor for epileptic fits. An increase level of vigilance is indicated (see Chapter 4).

A patient who faints regularly may have a phobia. Patients with a fear of needles frequently faint before or at injection. Equally, a patient who faints after treatment may be prone to postural hypotension. Such problems may be prevented by ensuring that patients return from a supine to a vertical position slowly after treatment.

Question 10

A history of rheumatic fever may indicate underlying valvular disease. There is no particular concern for the patient during treatment.

Question 11

Patients who suffer from diabetes mellitus need to have a regular pattern of food intake. Disruptions to the normal routine may make the patient liable to become hypoglycaemic (see Chapter 5).

Question 12

The chronic use of steroid medication can reduce the efficacy with which the pituitary–adrenal system responds to stress. There is little evidence to support the use of prophylactic steroid cover to prevent the occurrence of steroid crisis. This issue is dealt with in more detail in Chapter 5.

Question 13

Positive responses to this question may indicate that modification to the dental treatment is required to prevent postoperative haemorrhage.

Questions 14–16

These allow for the gleaning of information that is not covered elsewhere in the medical history questionnaire. The value of these questions will depend directly on the rigour to which positive answers are followed up in the dialogue history.

Readers are referred to the texts on the impact of medical conditions on dental treatment for a fuller account of the impact of medical history.

Physical evaluation of the dental patient

The physical evaluation of the patient is as important as the dialogue history. The combination of physical evaluation and past medical history will allow assessment of the patient's ability to tolerate treatment.

Physical evaluation is frequently underemphasized in dental practice in the UK. In other countries, more extensive physical evaluation is advocated.

As a minimum, the dentist should observe the patient. Such observation will allow the dentist to gain an overall impression of the patient. Such observations would include the patient's posture, body movements, speech, and skin.

Patient's posture

A patient who appears unnaturally stiff may be exhibiting signs of anxiety—a factor that may predispose to aggravation of pre-existing medical conditions.

A patient who claims not to be able to lie back in the chair may be anxious regarding treatment and feel threatened, or it may be a sign of heart failure, where the myocardium cannot cope with an increased venous return. Equally, in older patients, degenerative changes in the vertebral column may mean that it becomes physically impossible to extend the neck to achieve the normal posture required for dental treatment.

A useful question regarding the severity of symptoms induced when a patient is lying down is 'how many pillows do you use when you sleep?'. Patients who do not need more than two pillows do not have physical problems lying down.

Body movements

An anxious patient may fidget in the dental chair. Involuntary movements may be an indicator of underlying diseases; for example, a tremor may be seen in multiple sclerosis, hyperthroidism, or multiple sclerosis.

Quality of speech

A patient's anxiety may manifest itself in the way a patient talks. A patient who answers questions too quickly is often anxious about dental treatment. Nervousness may also manifest itself in a tremor in the voice.

Slurring of the speech may be the result of a pharmacological action from drugs such as alcohol. Some agents, particularly those used to control epilepsy, can cause a sluggish response. Patients who have had a stroke (cerebrovascular accident) may have difficulties in speech if that area of the brain was affected.

Feel of the patient's skin

If the dentist greets the patient by shaking hands, valuable insight can be obtained. A patient who is anxious will have a hand that feels cold and wet—sometimes described as like a piece of raw fish. Patients who are hyperthyroid or with diabetic acidosis will have hands that feel warm and dry.

Colour of the patient's skin

A patient's colour can also be a good diagnostic aid. Anxious patients will frequently have pale skin. Equally, pallor can be a manifestation of anaemia.

Cyanosis (a blue tinge to the skin—more obvious on the mucosa of the lips or in the nail beds) is a sign that the blood reaching those parts is poorly oxygenated. This can be for one of two reasons—either the lungs are not oxygenating the blood adequately or the heart is failing, or there is a congenital abnormality allowing oxygenated and deoxygenated blood to mix.

Jaundice (a yellow tinge to the skin or, more obviously, in the sclera of the eyes) may indicate past or indeed present liver disease.

Odours on the breath

During the dental examination, non-dental halitosis may be detected. This could be from alcohol used as an attempt to self medicate and provide anxiety relief. Other odours which may be detected include the fruity, sweet smell of acetone which is present during diabetic acidosis.

Rate and pattern of respiration

Healthy patients breathe between 10 and 20 times per minute. Breathing is shallow, silent, and does not involve the use of accessory muscles of respiration. A patient who is breathing rapidly may be hyperventilating due to panic.

Equally, patients who are making great efforts to breathe may have significantly compromised respiratory function. In such cases, it is important to establish how the observed pattern of breathing compares with the patient's normal function. Many patients with respiratory problems have 'good and bad days'. In such cases, treatment should be timed to coincide with the patient's 'good days'.

Special investigations

In the United Kingdom, the use of special investigations to provide further information on the patient's medical condition is rare.

Some authorities would recommend that all patients who are undergoing dental treatment should have their blood pressure recorded as part of the assessment process. A recent study has shown that a significant number of patients who attend for treatment have undiagnosed hypertension[6]. The inclusion of blood pressure measurement as a part of the assessment of patients receiving conscious sedation is now standard practice.

6 Kellog and Gobelli (2004) Hypertension in a dental school patient population. *J Dent Educ* **68**:956–964.

Preparation of the dental team

The attempts to prevent the occurrence of medical emergencies are not foolproof. The dental team should thus prepare to manage the unexpected.

The properly trained and equipped team treating an adequately assessed patient will be in the best position to manage complications should they occur. In view of the infrequency with which these events occur, it is not possible for the dental team to rely on experience to aid the management of these events and specific training is required.

Equipping the dental surgery

The equipment and drugs recommended for all dental practices are listed in Chapter 1 (pp. 7, 9). All areas where dentistry is carried out should have easy and rapid access to the drugs and equipment.

Preparation of the dental treatment environment

In order to have all drugs and emergency equipment available, the location of the emergency kit needs to be planned. It is impossible to be prescriptive about the location of such a kit other than to indicate that it must be available for use throughout the premises and be accessible.

Training of the dental team

Training in the management of medical emergencies is an integral part of the preparation process. In addition to being required by the General Dental Council[7], it is essential that any reduction in level of skill is compensated by regular training updates.

At the time of writing, the requirement is for all involved in the delivery of dental care to be competent at basic life support (see Chapter 9). Those involved in the provision of general anaesthesia or multiple-agent sedation are required to be competent at advanced life support (see Chapter 10).

It is recommended that all staff are trained in and can demonstrate competence in basic life support at least yearly and, preferably, at six-monthly intervals. Such training is best accomplished within the practice environment. It is recommended that the whole dental team should receive such training. All training in basic life support should be standardized for the team and conform to the Resuscitation Council guidelines. All members of staff should have a clear idea of how to work as a team, as well as being familiar with how to provide emergency care within their own working environment.

In addition to the formal regular training, staging mock emergencies serves to reinforce the skills that have been acquired and provide on-going training for staff. The regular practice of emergencies is also a requirement of the General Dental Council[7].

---

7 *Maintaining standards.* Guidance to dentists on professional and personal conduct, section 4.7. (Updated November 2001) General Dental Council, London.

Once the immediate medical emergency has been managed, patients may need to be transferred for further medical care. An important part of the preparation is to ensure that those whose duty it will be to summon assistance know both where to summon help from and also what information they will be required to give to ensure that the required help arrives promptly and at the correct location. Such information will include the clinical condition of the patient and a request for a paramedic ambulance rather than a patient transport ambulance. Ideally, a pre-filled proforma with the appropriate information should be kept adjacent to the telephone.

Summary

- Medical emergencies in the dental environment are a rare event. Their effect can be devastating for both the patient and the team treating them.
- Adequate assessment of the patient prior to treatment and the institution of appropriate anxiety management can reduce the likelihood of an emergency occurring.
- The dental team need to be prepared and trained to deal with untoward medical incidents in order to ensure the best possible outcome for the patient and also for those charged with their care.

Circulatory emergencies

Introduction

This chapter will highlight circulatory causes of collapse. The conditions covered are those in which the return of venous blood to the myocardium prevents the heart from maintaining a cardiac output which is compatible with a fully conscious state:

- Vasovagal attack (faint)
- Postural hypotension
- Anaphylactic shock.

All of these conditions have the potential to result in brain damage or death if measures are not taken to restore adequate cerebral perfusion. In the first two conditions, this is achieved with minimal treatment. The most serious of these conditions, both in terms of the treatment required and the potential outcome is anaphylactic shock.

Vasovagal attack

Diagnosis
- Light headed
- Warm
- Sweaty
- Pallor
- Slow pulse
- Loss of consciousness and collapse.

Exclusions
- Hypoglycaemia
- Other causes of collapse.

Immediate action
- Stop treatment
- Reassure patient
- Lie patient back—head down/feet up
- Loosen tight clothing
- Cool patient down.

Follow-up action
- Monitor pulse manually or with oximeter
- Oxygen via face mask
- Check blood sugar if possible
- If very prolonged, refer to emergency services.

Risk factors
- Anxiety
- Pain
- Fatigue
- Fasting
- More common in men than women
- Low blood pressure.

Diagnosis in the dental surgery

Diagnosis will depend on the presenting signs and symptoms as described above. The typical presentation is:
- Pale
- Sweaty
- Light headed.

Patients will usually recognize something is wrong. It is often not the first time they have experienced the sensations. In the pre-operative medical history, it is useful to ask about prior fainting experience. Often the highest risk is in those who have a habit of fainting. Other high-risk patients should be identified by the dental team early on (for example, young anxious men). Anxiety is clearly linked with fainting and irregular attenders and those in pain are often at risk.

Hypoglycaemia may be associated with fainting even in patients with no history of diabetes. If anxious patients starve themselves prior to treatment, the high circulating levels of epinephrine will mobilize glycogen stores in the liver. Once these stores are depleted the patient may complain of feeling faint. In these cases, hypoglycaemia is a contributing factor rather than the main loss of consciousness.

Patients will often faint after initial treatment, such as local anaesthetic injection, is complete. The relief of enduring the perceived 'worst' part of the treatment causes the vasovagal response as described above.

Patients will have low pulse rates (bradycardia) which will slowly recover on appropriate treatment. In response to the fall in blood pressure, the patient may then experience a tachycardia. Thus, it is common for patients to have a bradycardia when they lose consciousness, which then becomes a tachycardia once the venous return to the heart is increased by lying the patient down.

Immediate management

The key is to correct the cerebral hypoxia which is causing the light headedness and possible loss of consciousness. This is principally achieved by laying the patient back with their head down and their feet up. Dental chairs are usually ideal for this purpose and modern chairs can be preset to achieve a head down/feet up position quickly. This is the single most important treatment aspect for patients who have fainted.

Patients should be constantly reassured. As in all emergencies, this depends very clearly on the whole dental team. A calm, well-controlled team will be able to reassure a patient and often prevent any deterioration. Patients will feel very unwell and be embarrassed; they should be gently reassured throughout the incident. It is important they feel protected and private during a vulnerable time.

Monitoring is very useful and if a pulse oximeter is available, the pulse rate can give an indication of recovery. Alternatively, it is possible to monitor the pulse clinically. The pulse will be slow and perhaps challenging to feel at first. As the patient recovers, it will speed up and become stronger. In the recovery phase, patients will often describe their heart as pounding. This is a compensatory tachycardia which will settle quickly.

Drug treatment

As discussed in Chapter 1, oxygen is one of the required drugs for the treatment of emergencies in the dental surgery. It must be quickly available at the chairside with an appropriate delivery system. The cylinder must be checked regularly to ensure it is full. Oxygen is a very useful adjunct to treatment in those patients who have fainted and may aid recovery.

Whether or not to abandon treatment

The vast majority of faints are self-limiting and patients will recover without further incident. However, they should not be underestimated and it may be appropriate to abandon treatment for the day.

The treating dentist must be aware that by abandoning the treatment for the day it is possible to condition patients that fainting prevents dental treatment progressing. Abandoning the treatment may increase the likelihood of fainting at subsequent visits and thus, if possible, the treatment should proceed.

Use of sedation

A mature discussion with the patient outlining what steps are still required and alternatives may be useful both in reassuring them and in deciding on a future treatment plan. Sedation is a useful adjunct in patients prone to fainting and could be discussed at this stage. Even nitrous oxide/oxygen inhalation sedation can have a profound effect on a patient's anxiety—enough to deal with the possibility of fainting. This makes the whole visit easier on both the patient and on the dental team.

Prolonged fainting

In prolonged faints, seizures may occur which can be confused with epilepsy. This usually occurs in patients in whom immediate management has been slow. Management is the same as above. In very prolonged faints, hospital admission should be considered.

Post-recovery management

On recovery, the administration of oral glucose is a popular treatment. This can elevate the patient's blood sugar and thus prevent hypoglycaemia causing a second vasovagal event. Administering high concentrations of glucose may cause nausea and vomiting. Glucose is better used as a prophylactic measure, where it is administered before treatment to patients who have not eaten prior to treatment.

In patients who give a history of fainting, pre-treatment instructions should include specific advice to eat before they attend.

Postural hypotension

Diagnosis
- Light headed on standing, after lying for a long period
- Light headed after short walk, after lying for a long period
- Other symptoms of a vasovagal attack.

Exclusions
- Hypoglycaemia
- Other causes of collapse.

Immediate action
- Reassure patient
- Lie patient back—head down/feet up
- Loosen tight clothing
- Cool patient down.

Follow-up action
- Monitor pulse manually or with oximeter
- Oxygen via face mask
- Check blood sugar if possible
- If very prolonged, refer to emergency services
- Return patient to the vertical very slowly and in stages.

Risk factors
- Medication:
  - anti-hypertensive medication
  - phenothiaside medication
  - tricyclic antidepressants
  - narcotics
  - anti-Parkinson drugs.
- Prolonged periods in a supine position
- Inadequate postural reflex:
  - pregnancy
  - old age.
- Inadequate venous return:
  - varicose veins
- Physical exhaustion
- Low blood pressure.

Diagnosis in the dental surgery
Diagnosis depends on the presence of the presenting signs. There are two typical scenarios:
1. The patient has received dental treatment for a significant time period and complains of feeling faint when they try to stand up.
2. A patient gets up and walks from the dental chair to the reception desk to make an appointment but feels faint when they stop walking.

Postural hypotension can be defined as a disorder of the autonomic nervous system in which syncope occurs when the patient assumes the vertical position. It varies in a number of important ways from vasovagal syncope:

- Seldom associated with fear and anxiety
- Caused by a drop in systolic blood pressure of at least 20mmHg
- Usually a predisposing factor or a history of repeated events, such as feeling faint when getting up from sleep.

Immediate management

The key is to correct the cerebral hypoxia which is causing the light headedness and possible loss of consciousness. This is principally achieved by laying the patient back with their head down and their feet up. In this respect, the management is similar to that for a vasovagal syncope. Once the patient has recovered, they should be returned to the vertical position slowly and in approximately three stages, with sufficient time allowed at each stage for any dizziness to pass.

Once standing, the patient should be allowed to stand in the surgery, adjacent to the dental chair, for two minutes to ensure that postural hypotension does not subsequently develop. Allowing the patient to walk from the surgery may mask a poor venous return, as the muscle pump in the legs will increase venous return. When the patient stops walking, they may feel light headed again.

Prevention and long-term management

The best management of postural hypotension is to prevent the symptoms. The medical history as described in Chapter 2 provides the tools for diagnosis. If patients indicate they have a tendency to feel faint on rising, then as a precaution, the treating dentist should always adopt the three-stage approach to returning the patient to a vertical position after treatment.

If the symptoms of postural hypotension suddenly develop, the advice of the patient's GP should be sought.

Anaphylactic shock

Diagnosis
- Presentation varies widely
- Erythema of face
- Itching
- Oedema
- Wheeze
- Loss of consciousness
- Weak and rapid pulse
- Blood pressure low and may be difficult to record.

Exclusions
- Anaphylactic reaction rather than full-blown 'shock'
- Other causes of collapse.

Immediate management
- Stop treatment
- Seek help
- Talk to patient
- Lie patient flat with legs raised
- Administer high-flow oxygen via face mask
- 0.5–1mg adrenaline intramuscularly
- Monitor clinically and electronically if possible
- Repeat adrenaline every 60 seconds if no or limited response
- Arrange hospital admission.

Delayed management
- Continued adrenaline
- Antihistamine and steroid treatment
- Intravenous fluids
- Possible intubation.

Risk factors
- Atopic individuals—asthma, eczema, hay fever
- Contact with common allergens—latex, penicillins.

Diagnosis in the dental surgery

The word anaphylaxis literally means 'lack of protection' as opposed to prophylaxis which means 'protection'. This definition helps in an understanding of what happens to the body's systems during anaphylactic shock.

Anaphylactic shock is the endpoint of a systemic allergic reaction. It is part of a continuum from simple angioedema, such as lip swelling, thorough self-limiting anaphylactic reactions characterized by some of the above symptoms. Patients may have erythema and swelling but no wheeze, for example.

Full anaphylactic shock is characterized by circulatory and respiratory collapse:
- Blood pressure plummets
- Airways become increasingly closed
- Patients become distressed and collapse, losing consciousness.

Risk assessment

As with all medical emergencies, preparation is the key and the first rule of preparation is risk assessment of the patient and the environment. Common allergens encountered in the dental environment include latex (gloves, rubber dam, etc.) and drugs (penicillins, etc.). It is important to include questions about previous allergic reactions in a pre-operative medical history. Any previous reactions to potential allergens should be taken very seriously and not discounted unless the operator is sure there is an alternative explanation. Alternatives are becoming available for latex products and there is a convincing school of thought that says dental surgeries should move as quickly as possible to be latex free.

Increasingly, patients are becoming more aware of allergies in general, particularly food allergies. The most common life-threatening example is peanuts and, although this is not commonly encountered in the dental environment directly, there is some evidence that patients with proven allergies may be more susceptible to others. Again, risk assessment is vital.

Immediate management

Treatment varies according to severity but there should be no hesitation if there is any doubt—adrenaline is life-saving in those having anaphylactic shock.

Treatment depends on the swift and efficient delivery of adrenaline into the circulation. This is most efficiently achieved by the intramuscular injection of 0.5–1mg into the deltoid muscle in the upper arm. All patients who reach this stage of management will require hospital admission and continued monitoring.

The more difficult treatment group are those who have mild reactions without breathing difficulties or circulatory collapse. These patients may have isolated swelling around their lips, for example, where they have come into contact with latex products. Since antihistamines are not a required emergency drug in the dental surgery, the advice for these patients is to continue to monitor them in case of deterioration but to get them to hospital as quickly as possible. There, antihistamines can be administered promptly. Obviously, this patient will move into a higher risk category for future care.

Delayed management

Adrenaline doses may have to be continued for some time in prolonged cases. Antihistamines and steroids may be given intravenously in hospital to aid long-term recovery.

After recovery, attempts should be made to identify the allergen which led to the reaction. This will involve referral to an allergy clinic for testing. Allergen avoidance will be instituted along with the provision of an Epipen® to the patient in case of further emergencies.

Central nervous system emergencies

Introduction

This chapter will deal with emergencies originating in the central nervous system (CNS). The conditions covered are:
- Epilepsy
- Stroke (cerebrovascular accident)
- Transient ischaemic attack (TIA).

Epilepsy

Epilepsy is actually a catch-all term for a number of distinct conditions and syndromes with causes ranging from hereditary to unknown. The definition that is generally recognized is 'a chronic brain disorder of various aetiologies characterized by recurrent seizures due to excessive discharge of cerebral neurons'. For the dental surgeon, the intricacies of the individual diagnosis are unimportant but the ability to recognize and promptly deal with the seizures is vital. The manifestations of the condition range from short absences, where the patient may appear not to be paying attention, through to 'grand mal' fits.

Diagnosis
- Usually known epileptic
- Varied presentation
- Simple vacancy, through petit mal, to full grand mal seizure
- Varied duration.

Immediate management
- Stop treatment
- Ensure safety of patient and team
- Maintain airway
- Monitor length and strength of seizure
- Reassure
- High-flow oxygen via face mask.

Risk factors
- Usually history of seizures
- Stress
- Pain
- Infection.

Delayed management
- If prolonged and/or recurring (status epilepticus), seek hospital admission
- Intranasal midazolam
- If first seizure, then cause must be investigated.

Diagnosis in the dental surgery

Seizures can occur for a multitude of reasons in the dental surgery. As described in Chapter 3, they can simply be the result of a prolonged faint. Other seizures commonly seen in the dental surgery are usually the result of epilepsy or epileptic syndromes. Patients will usually give a history of seizures in the past.

Patients will often, but not always, report a prodromal phase when they are aware that they are going to seizure. Prompt action at this point may avert injury to the patient and the dental team.

Seizures may be simply evidenced by a short loss of awareness which will be self-limiting. The classic tonic-clonic seizure can be of varied strength and length. The majority will be short and self-limiting.

Prevention

The best management of seizures in the dental surgery is to prevent the seizure. This is frequently easier to say than to achieve.

Patients often understand their disease very well and respond well to questioning about risk factors. Reduction of anxiety is a key feature of prevention.

Risk assessment

The most important aspect of prevention is once again risk assessment. A thorough medical history is vital and will reveal details of the patient's epilepsy history which the dental team will need to take into account when assessing the risk of treatment. Factors to note include:

- Drug therapy—drug type, drug dose, drug frequency, length of use
- Treating physician—neurologist or a GP?
- Causes of previous seizures—pain, anxiety, etc.
- Seizure history—has it been three years or three days since last seizure and seizure type? Is there a prodromal phase? Has there ever been status epilepticus?.

These questions will allow the team to assess how likely a seizure is for this individual patient and to take appropriate measures to limit the risk and be prepared to treat any seizures which may occur.

Sedation

It is vital to reduce the risk as far as possible. If a patient reports that seizures worsen as a result of anxiety, it may be appropriate to consider some form of anxiety control such as sedation, either inhalation or intravenous.

When considering the use of sedation, it is important to remember that hypoxia is a potential trigger for epileptic fits. When intravenous sedation is used, a wise precaution is the administration of supplemental oxygen via nasal cannulae.

Preventing injury

A rubber mouth prop may be used when treating patients who are prone to fitting. The mouth prop will not prevent the fit occurring, but it will help prevent injury to the dental team as a result of the patient biting during a fit.

Immediate management

The first priority is the safety of the patient and the dental team. There is no point in having two emergencies to deal with instead of one. Treatment should be stopped at the first sign of difficulty. This may be the patient reporting something—they often have very good insight into seizure progression. It is important to note, however, that not all patients report a prodromal stage. Seizures can occur dramatically and unannounced.

Patients should be allowed to seizure freely with the removal of any objects from the area which may hurt them. The airway should be maintained if it is safe to do so and oxygen may be administered. The dental team should not put itself in danger by trying to take out anything in the patient's mouth etc. Intervention should be limited to airway maintenance.

A useful adjunct to treatment is oxygen therapy and this can be safely given via a face mask. Fitting patients use a higher amount of oxygen than those who are not fitting. Ventilation may also be compromised by the fit activity. This will lead to hypoxia, which may precipatate further fitting.

Recovery phase

Recovery can vary widely. Some patients will recover very quickly and show little lasting consequences. More commonly, the patient will be slow to recover and be very tired for some time afterwards. Treatment will not be completed that day and discussion of future plans should be postponed. It is vital that the patient feels secure, protected, and not embarrassed in the dental setting, so they must be dealt with very sympathetically throughout. Reassurance in the immediate post-seizure phase is very helpful.

Follow-up

Follow-up care will depend on the history and severity of the seizure but, if in any doubt, medical help should be sought. It is particularly important that medical help is sought if the fit is unusual for the patient in severity, duration, or provoking factor. Any patient who fits and has no previous history must be sent for urgent investigation.

Delayed treatment

If fitting is very prolonged (longer than five minutes) or recurring seizures occur, this is classed as status epilepticus and the patient requires immediate emergency hospital admission. Cerebral damage can occur if this is delayed. The patient will be given anti-seizure medication in the accident and emergency department.

Stroke (cerebrovascular accident)

The brain needs around 20% of the total blood volume at any time. If this blood flow is interrupted for even a short time, then neurone death and brain ischaemia are a risk. There are two principle types of stroke:
- Ischaemic strokes occur as a result of blood vessel occlusion
- Haemorrhagic strokes occur as a result of blood vessel rupture.

Diagnosis
- Can be difficult to diagnosis
- Signs and symptoms can be subtle
- Confusion
- Muscle weakness
- Inability to speak
- Loss of consciousness.

Immediate management
- Stop treatment
- Establish level of consciousness
- Maintain airway if necessary
- High-flow oxygen via face mask
- Arrange immediate transfer to hospital
- Reassure patient
- Monitor patient.

Exclusions
- Faint
- Other CNS emergencies.

Risk factors
- Elderly
- More common in men than women
- Hypertension
- Smoking
- Obesity
- Ischaemic heart disease (e.g. angina)
- Previous stroke.

Diagnosis in the dental surgery

This can be a very difficult diagnosis to make. The symptoms can range from apparent mild confusion, through loss of speech, to a full stroke causing immediate collapse and possibly cardiac arrest.

Dentists are not expected to know the details of stroke diagnosis other than to have a low threshold of suspicion and seek help quickly. No sign or symptom should be ignored and clinicians should have a particularly low threshold of suspicion in the high-risk groups. Strokes occur most commonly in the elderly, with men at greater risk than women.

The difficulty in diagnosis due to the wide variation in clinical effects can present a problem for the dental team. A false positive diagnosis, where management is initiated for a patient who has not had a stroke is better than a false negative where a patient who has suffered a stroke receives no treatment.

Stroke has the basic risk pattern of other ischaemic disease. Although simplified, it is useful to think of those at risk of a myocardial infarction as also at risk of a stroke. This includes:

• Smoking
• Obesity
• Hypertension
• Diabetes.

A previous stroke significantly increases the patient's risk and a careful medical history should pick this up.

Management

Dental treatment should be stopped immediately. Patients may show immediate weakness on one side of their body, most easily seen on the face by the dental surgeon. This is not to be confused with the temporary phenomenon of facial nerve paralysis after local anaesthetic injection. Patients may not be able to communicate.

In some cases, patients may be completely unable to speak; in others, patients may be able to speak but may be unable to recall certain words. In such situations, when talking, the patient may pause and be apparently searching for words. In more extreme cases, patients may lose consciousness and the airway must be maintained as a priority. Oxygen should be given via a face mask.

Prompt transfer to hospital is the key. Mortality and morbidity can be significantly reduced with immediate assessment and care in the form of a specialist stroke team.

Patients should be reassured and their condition should be explained. They will be very apprehensive and will benefit from a well-managed approach to their care. It should be emphasized that help will be sought very promptly.

The patient should be maintained in a comfortable position. If the blood pressure is raised and the patient is conscious, they should be maintained with the head slightly above the heart. The use of sedative agents is to be discouraged.

It is also vital to have members of the team to deal with any family members who may be present. The relatives will inevitably be concerned and may wish to be with the patient. It is important that, prior to them seeing the patient, they receive an explanation of what has occurred, as well as what to expect when they see their relative.

Transient ischaemic attack

Transient ischaemic attacks (TIAs) are self-limiting, temporary events caused by non-permanent interruption to the cerebral perfusion. TIAs may be an early warning of a full stroke.

TIAs normally last for between 2 and 10 minutes. They have been described as being as short as 10 seconds or as long as 1 hour.

Diagnosis
- Can be difficult to diagnosis
- Clinical signs depend on area of the brain affected
- Transient numbness or weakness of the legs or arms
  - may be described as 'pins and needles'
- Transient monocular blindness
  - black or grey shadow spreading and receding over all or part of the visual field of one eye
- Consciousness often unimpared
- Thought processes slowed.

Immediate management
- Stop treatment
- Establish level of consciousness
- Maintain airway if necessary
- High-flow oxygen via face mask
- Reassure patient
- Monitor patient
- Arrange for transfer to hospital.

Exclusions
Other CNS emergencies.

Risk factors
- As for a cerebrovascular accident (CVA)
- Patient who has regular TIAs.

Diagnosis in the dental surgery
As with a CVA, the diagnosis of a TIA can be extremely difficult. It can also be difficult to distinguish between a CVA and a TIA.

In the case of a TIA, if the patient gives a history of having such episodes, the effects that the episodes have had on the patient can give a good guide, as the symptoms in a particular patient tend to be consistent.

If any of the symptoms described above are present, then the emergency medical services should be called. In patients who have no previous history of a CVA or TIA, a first TIA may be a warning sign of a CVA, particularly if it lasts for more than an hour.

Management
The management of the TIA is essentially the same as for a CVA. Even if the patient has a regular history of TIAs, it is wise to seek emergency medical help. If, after assessment, it is decided that hospitalization is not required, the patient should not drive home, and should be accompanied by a responsible adult.

Endocrine emergencies

Introduction

This chapter will deal with emergencies originating from problems with the body's endocrine systems. Conditions included are:

- Hypoglycaemia
- Hyperglycaemia
- Adrenal crisis.

Hypoglycaemia

Diagnosis
- Usually known diabetic
- Rapid onset of collapse
- Confusion
- Aggression
- Sweaty
- Palpitations
- Tremor
- Headache
- Drowsiness
- Pallor
- Loss of consciousness.

Immediate management
- Stop treatment
- Lie flat
- If conscious—oral glucose
- If unconscious—1mg glucagon intramuscularly
- Monitor consciousness
- Reassure patient
- Consider hospital admission.

Risk factors
- Diabetes
- Excess insulin or missed meal
- Anxiety
- Infection
- Alcohol consumption
- Other systemic illness.

Delayed management
- If prolonged or first attack, then hospital admission essential
- Diabetic management may require review.

Diagnosis in the dental surgery
Figures suggest that hypoglycaemia affects around 20% of diabetics at least once a year, usually as a result of poor control either acutely or chronically. It occurs when too much insulin or oral antidiabetic medication is taken, not enough food is eaten, or from a sudden increase in the amount of exercise without an increase in food intake. Risk assessment is vital, as described in Chapter 2. Although hypoglycaemia can rarely occur in non-diabetics, it is much more commonly seen in the diabetic population. The other group of the population who can become acutely hypoglycaemic are those suffering from anorexia nervosa.

Diabetics must be assessed fully using a pre-operative history. This should include:
- A history of drug therapy
- Hospital admissions
- Previous hypoglycaemic attacks
- Information about treating physicians.

It is useful to get some idea of glucose control from the patient. It may be necessary to liaise with the treating physician, particularly if undertaking extensive treatment which might interfere with the patient's ability to maintain normal dietary habits.

Patients will usually understand their disease very well and be aware of early symptoms. They will often ask for sugar or even have some with them. These requests should not be ignored or delayed in any circumstances.

Patients will appear pale and sweaty; they will often seem confused and subsequently lose consciousness. Initial symptoms may be confused with a simple faint. However, the patient will not recover when simple measures, such as lying down flat, are instituted. The dental team should treat all faints in diabetics as very suspicious. Oral glucose is not going to do these patients any harm when they are still conscious and able to swallow. It is useful to catch the symptoms as early as possible since treatment is much simpler in the conscious patient.

Liaison with the treating physician can be crucially important in risk assessment of diabetic patients. They often know a great deal about the glucose control of individual patients and can be useful sources of advice.

Patients will become gradually more and more disorientated and eventually lose consciousness.

Immediate management

The conscious patient

Treatment depends on the prompt provision of glucose. This can be in the form of liquid, tablets, or gels if the patient is conscious. Patients, particularly those who are poorly controlled, will often carry a form of sugar with them. It is important to have an alternative source available in the dental surgery such as glucose tablets, glucose powder, or high-sugar drinks. Proprietary gels are available for purchase which provide a useful way of ensuring high doses of glucose enter the patient's circulation as quickly as possible. The substances are used for similar purposes by high-performance athletes, such as cyclists, to obtain important energy boosts.

The unconscious patient

If the patient is unconscious, then the solution is not as simple. It is impossible to give oral glucose and, therefore, intramuscular glucagon should be administered. This is an essential emergency drug in the dental surgery and comes in a prepared form ready to inject. Administration of glucagon pharmacologically leads to a rapid rise in blood glucose, hence injectable glucagon is an appropriate pharmacological treatment for hypoglycaemia. The deltoid muscle in the upper arm is a convenient place for this injection.

As in all loss of consciousness situations, it is vital to maintain the patient's airway. The provision of oxygen via a face mask is also recommended.

Delayed treatment

Slow recovery or unconscious patients require hospital transfer for accurate blood glucose measurement and appropriate treatment.

Hyperglycaemia

Hyperglycaemia is very rare and occurs in known diabetics after inadequate or absent insulin administration. It is very unlikely to present in the dental surgery.

Diagnosis
- Poorly controlled insulin-dependent diabetic
- Missed insulin
- Often been ill for days
- Nausea and vomiting
- Slow to collapse
- Abdominal pain
- Drowsy
- Characteristic smell of fruit or sweet breath
- Rapid weak pulse
- Normal to low blood pressure.

Exclusions
- Hypoglycaemia
- Faint
- Central nervous system emergency.

Immediate management
- Stop treatment
- Reassure
- Airway management, if necessary
- Hospital transfer.

Delayed management
- Blood sugar measurement
- Insulin
- Monitor
- Consider reviewing diabetic management.

Diagnosis in the dental surgery

Hyperglycaemia is a much rarer occurrence than hypoglycaemia. It does not produce sudden loss of consciousness and patients are often ill for some time. They are much more likely to present to their treating physician or diabetic management team.

The most common cause of hyperglycaemia in diabetics is one or more missed insulin doses. It is, therefore, almost uniquely encountered in type 1 diabetics. It can also occur as a result of changes in dietary habits, stress, less exercise than normal, and other illness such as flu.

Symptoms of hyperglycaemia are the same as those of untreated diabetes. They do not appear suddenly, but over a period of time. They include:
- Tiredness
- Frequent urination
- Thirst.

If symptoms are prolonged, they can cause weight loss and blurred vision.

In the long term, hyperglycaemia can increase the likelihood of complications of diabetes, such as damage to the kidneys, eyes, and nerves of the feet, heart disease, and circulation problems in the extremities.

Treatment

Signs and symptoms of hyperglycaemia picked up during the history or treatment in the dental environment require prompt referral to a physician. The patient will almost certainly have a treating team of diabetic professionals. Liaison with this team is essential to prevent further deterioration. The patient will require long-term management of their diabetes and may need their insulin regimen adjusted.

Adrenal crisis

Adrenal insufficiency is seen in patients when the adrenal cortex produces insufficient cortisol for physiological demands. Except in specific conditions, such as Addison's disease, it very rarely progresses to collapse.

Diagnosis

- Can be over many days or acute response to stress
- Rapid weak pulse
- Hypotension
- Pallor
- Loss of consciousness.

Risk factors

- Adrenal disease (e.g. Addison's)
- Dehydration
- Long-term steroid use
- Stress
- Systemic illness.

Exclusions

Faint.

Immediate treatment

- Stop treatment
- High-flow oxygen via face mask
- Lie flat with feet up
- Reassure
- Monitor consciousness
- Airway management, if necessary
- Monitor blood pressure, if possible
- Arrange hospital transfer.

Delayed management

- intravenous steroids
- intravenous fluids
- investigation of cause.

Diagnosis in the dental surgery

This condition is one that is frequently taught in the dental environment, but never seen. There is a theoretical risk that the long-term use of steroid medication decreases the body's ability to produce steroid at times of stress. This lack of steroid precipitates the crisis. The condition was originally described in cardio-thoracic surgery, where the operative stress is much greater than in routine dentistry!

Adrenal crisis is a very rare but life-threatening condition requiring prompt doses of intravenous corticosteroids to replace the absent physiological response. Patients will usually have been sick for some days, often with other systemic illness, but adrenal crisis can occur acutely as a result of a psychologically or physiologically stressful episode.

Glucocorticoids are secreted by the adrenal glands and are non-specific cardiac stimulants that activate release of vasoactive substances. The adrenal medullae normally secrete 80% epinephrine and 20% norepinephrine. Sympathetic stimulation results in secretion. The adrenal cortex produces cortisol, aldosterone, and androgens. In the absence of corticosteroids, stress can result in hypotension, shock, and death.

Adrenal insufficiency can be described as primary or secondary.

Primary adrenal insufficiency

Primary adrenal insufficiency may be caused by the destruction of the gland. This destruction can have various causes, including:

- Infection
- Neoplasia
- Haemorrhage.

However, the most frequent cause is idiopathic atrophy, which is thought to be autoimmune in origin. Primary adrenal insufficiency may also be caused by metabolic failure (e.g. insufficient hormone production). This failure may be a result of:

- Congenital adrenal hyperplasia
- Enzyme inhibitors
- Cytotoxic agents.

Primary adrenocortical insufficiency is rare and it can occur at any age.

Secondary adrenal insufficiency

Secondary adrenal insufficiency can be caused by hypopituitarism due to hypothalamic–pituitary disease, or it may result from suppression of the hypothalamic–pituitary axis by exogenous steroids. It is relatively common; extensive therapeutic use of steroids has increased the incidence.

Prophylactically covering at-risk patients with pre-operative steroids is controversial but some authorities recommend increased oral doses or intramuscular supplementation prior to treatment. There is little or no evidence for such a recommendation. Others suggest increased monitoring, such as blood pressure, and the availability of intravenous steroids may be appropriate.

Diagnosis can be difficult due to the vagueness of signs and symptoms. There should be a low threshold of suspicion in patients in the at-risk groups and any collapse should be promptly assessed.

Management

Since intravenous steroids are not a required drug in the dental surgery, it is not appropriate to institute any treatment other than reassurance and prompt referral if adrenal crisis is suspected. If the patient loses consciousness, oxygen therapy and airway protection should be instituted.

Prompt transfer to hospital where intravenous corticosteroids and fluids can be delivered is the key.

Respiratory emergencies

This chapter will highlight respiratory causes of emergencies, covering the following conditions:
- Hyperventilation
- Asthma
- Upper airway obstruction.

Hyperventilation

Hyperventilation occurs when ventilation is increased above the normal metabolic requirements. It should be more appropriately called 'hyper-ventilation syndrome'. It is described in an acute and chronic form. We are concerned here with the acute form since this can present as a medical emergency, particularly in stressful situations. The chronic form has similar signs and symptoms but they are much more subtle in their presentation and are often confused with other conditions. There is some evidence that it is a very underdiagnosed condition.

Diagnosis
- Fast breathing
- Occurs in around 10% of the population at some time
- Most common in young women
- Anxious
- Wweak
- Light headed
- Dizzy
- Paraesthesia of extremities and peri-oral region
- Tetany
- Tremors
- Somach pain
- Nausea and vomiting
- Fast pulse (tachycardia)
- Chest pain
- Palpitations.

Risk factors
- Anxiety
- Pain
- Previous episodes
- Cardiovascular disease.

Immediate management
- Stop treatment
- Reassure
- Reduce anxiety
- Encouraging re-breathing of carbon dioxide via bag or cupped hands.

Delayed management
- In prolonged cases, consider anxiolytics such as nitrous oxide
- Consider future treatment with sedation.

Diagnosis in dental surgery

Acute hyperventilation is very common, particularly in stress-inducing environments such as the dental surgery. It is characterized by:

- Fast, shallow, gulping breathing
- Often accompanied by panic and tears.

It progresses to:

- Tetany
- Paraesthesia
- Even to loss of consciousness.

It occurs more commonly in patients who are anxious and/or in pain.

Presentation is often very dramatic. Patients show a variety of signs and symptoms including:

- Agitation
- Hyperpnea and tachypnea
- Chest pain
- Dyspnea
- Wheezing
- Dizziness
- Palpitations
- Tetanic cramps (carpopedal spasm)
- Paraesthesias (often peri-oral)
- Generalized weakness
- Syncope.

In extreme cases, the patient can lose consciousness.

Immediate management

The key to management is reduction of anxiety. This is principally accomplished by reassurance and getting the patients to breathe more slowly. Re-breathing of carbon dioxide may be necessary to redress the metabolic imbalance created by the fast breathing. This re-breathing is traditionally done by asking the patient to breath in and out of a paper bag, hence re-breathing their own expired carbon dioxide. The same outcome can be more simply and less dramatically achieved by simply asking the patient to clasp their hands around their mouth and take slow, deep breaths. This again will allow them to breath a mixture of 'new' air and their own expired breath. It has also been suggested that using a paper bag can have the advantage that the movements of the bag can be used as a feedback mechanism. The patient is asked to make the bag movements greater and slower until a normal pattern of breathing is achieved.

The safety of these techniques has been questioned in the literature and some authorities suggest that the risk of hypoxia is greater than the benefit achieved. They suggest that reassurance, explanation, with possible acute sedation with benzodiazepines are a more appropriate group of treatment measures.

Asking the patient to exhale fully, with physical compression of the upper thorax may allow a 'fuller' breath to be achieved. Patients with hyperventilation often use only the upper thorax and have hyperinflated lungs throughout the respiratory cycle. Because the residual lung volume is high, the patient is unable to take a full tidal volume and experiences dyspnea.

Long-term management

Prevention depends on the identification of the at-risk groups. Previous attacks are a very good indication that extra caution should be taken and perhaps sedation should be considered.

Explanation of the cause, physiology, and treatment to a susceptible patient can often be enough to prevent further attacks. Treatment in a calming environment by a sympathetic team who demonstrate control can reassure the at-risk patient.

The use of relaxation techniques, where breathing is controlled, has also been recommended as an appropriate management technique.

Asthma

Asthma is a very common disease in the population. It is characterized by increased airway reactivity to allergens or other stimuli such as drugs, causing:
- Narrowing of the airways
- Associated wheeze
- Respiratory distress.

Acute attacks tend to occur in the poorly controlled and occur intermittently.

Diagnosis
- Usually known asthmatics
- Expiratory wheeze
- Cough
- Rapid pulse
- Hypertension
- Panic
- Anxiety and distress
- Shallow breathing.

Risk factors
- Stress
- Exposure to allergens (e.g. latex)
- Other systemic illness
- Poor control.

Immediate management
- Stop treatment
- Reassure
- Stress reduction
- High-flow oxygen via face mask
- Inhaled salbutamol (two puffs initially)—patient will usually carry their own
- Monitor condition and consciousness
- Continue salbutamol.

Delayed management
- Continued salbutamol
- Hospital transfer for nebulized salbutamol
- In prolonged cases, intravenous salbutamol and intravenous steroids may be necessary.

Diagnosis in the dental surgery
Asthma is one of the most common diseases encountered in the dental surgery, particularly amongst the young. The vast majority of asthmatics are well controlled with inhaled corticosteroids and occasional 'rescue' medication such as salbutamol. Attacks are therefore rare.

Asthmatics have acute episodes when the air passages in their lungs become narrower, and breathing becomes more difficult. These problems are caused by an oversensitivity of the lungs and airways. The lungs and airways can overreact to certain triggers causing:
- The lining of the airways to become inflamed and swollen
- Tightening of the muscles that surround the airways
- Increased production of mucus.

Breathing becomes harder and may hurt. This is usually accompanied by coughing, wheezing, or whistling from the lungs. Wheezing occurs because of the rush of air which moves through the narrowed airways.

Risk assessment is again vital in the prevention of attacks. A careful history will reveal much about the patient's asthma history. The following information is all vital:
- Drug therapy
- Dose and frequency of medication
- Previous attacks
- Previous hospital admissions
- Potential triggers.

Patients may have different and varied triggers. These can include:
- Allergens such as pollen or house dust
- Respiratory infections
- Airway irritants such as air pollution or strong perfumes
- Exercise
- Stress
- Smoke
- Drug therapy.

Aspirin and other non-steroidal anti-inflammatory drugs can exacerbate asthma and have been implicated in around 20% of acute attacks. Care should be taken when prescribing to asthmatics to avoid potential problems.

When an acute attack does occur, it is usually in the uncontrolled or severely asthmatic and often associated with a stressful episode. Patients will struggle for breath, wheeze, and cough. They will instinctively look for their salbutamol and should receive it immediately.

Immediate management

A combination of reassurance, inhaled salbutamol, and oxygen will be sufficient to deal with the vast majority of incidents. Prolonged cases (so-called 'status asthmaticus') require immediate transfer to hospital for systemic bronchodilators and steroid therapy. Asthma can be life-threatening and should not be underestimated despite its common occurrence.

Treatment should be stopped immediately and the patient should be placed in a comfortable position. This usually means sitting the patient up. It has also been suggested that asking the patient to stand with their back against a wall may be of benefit. Standing upright encourages deeper breathing than if the patient is bent forward. They should be reassured in a calm controlled voice. They will understand usually what is happening but they will find it difficult not to panic because of the difficulty in breathing. Oxygen should be given in an attempt to prevent hypoxia caused by the shallow breathing.

Salbutamol should be administered as quickly as possible; depending on the severity of the attack the patient may be capable of using their inhaler as normal. If not, then they should be assisted. If conventional inhaler use proves difficult, then multiple puffs can be expressed into an appropriate 'spacer' and the patient can breathe from that. Overdose with inhaled salbutamol is not a risk; it is more important to get the bronchodilator into the airways.

Long-term management

In prolonged cases, hospital referral is vital. Patients will require systemic bronchodilators and steroids. They will also require review of their prevention regimen.

1400 people die in the UK each year from asthma-associated complications. Dental teams must know how to deal promptly with any acute problems and refer when necessary.

Upper airway obstruction

Upper airway obstruction due to blockage is usually preventable but can inevitably occur in the dental patient. Care must always be taken when using instruments in a patient's mouth and the judicious use of rubber dam and mouth sponges is vital to prevent the potentially serious consequences of upper airway obstruction.

Diagnosis
- Coughing
- Holding throat
- Often during treatment, when something has obviously dropped or dislodged
- Gasping breaths
- Rising pulse
- Stridor if partial blockage
- Silence if complete blockage.

Risk factors
- Supine patients
- Intricate dentistry with small instruments
- Poor suction
- Lack of rubber dam or mouth sponge.

Immediate management
- Stop treatment
- Suction at back of mouth if visible blockage
- Sit patient up
- Encourage coughing
- Five firm back slaps between shoulder blades
- Five firm abdominal thrusts (Heimlich manoeuvre)
- Repeat back slaps and abdominal thrusts until blockage is dislodged
- Seek help
- Emergency hospital admission if prolonged.

Delayed treatment
- Possible cricothyroid puncture to allow breathing
- Laryngoscopy
- Bronchoscopy.

Diagnosis in the dental surgery
It is usually fairly acute and obvious when an upper airway becomes blocked in a patient. The dentist will often be aware of a dropped instrument or dislodged root which has caused the problem. Patients will immediately cough and their hands will instinctively move to their throat.

Avoidance is better than treatment and, therefore, everything should be done to prevent the rare but real risk of inhaled foreign bodies. Rubber dam should be used whenever possible and both dentist and dental nurse should be constantly vigilant. High-volume suction can protect patients during treatment and the appropriate use of sponges can be helpful.

Even with the most elaborate protection, the obvious problem of effectively working in part of the patient's airway can lead to problems. Foreign bodies can lodge it any part of the airway depending on shape, size, and treatment.

Immediate management

The majority of cases will be resolved after a bout of vigorous coughing. Large items will not be able to travel far and will cause instant reaction as the patient sits upright and coughs vigorously. Smaller items may lodge further down the airways and prove more stubborn.

More stubborn blockages will require a combination of back slaps and abdominal thrusts. The UK Resuscitation Council have produced guidelines on the sequence to be followed:

1. If blockage of the airway is only partial, the victim will usually be able to clear it by coughing, but if obstruction is complete, urgent intervention is required to prevent asphyxia.
2. If the victim is conscious and breathing, despite evidence of obstruction:
- Encourage them to continue coughing but do nothing else.
3. If the victim is conscious and obstruction is complete or the victim shows signs of exhaustion or becomes cyanosed:
- Carry out back blows:
  - Remove any obvious debris or loose teeth from the mouth.
  - Stand to the side and slightly behind them.
  - Support their chest with one hand and lean the victim well forwards so that when the obstructing object is dislodged it comes out of the mouth rather than goes further down the airway.
  - Give up to five sharp blows between the scapulae (shoulder blades) with the heel of your other hand; each blow should be aimed at relieving the obstruction, so all five need not necessarily be given.
- If the back blows fail, carry out abdominal thrusts:
  - Stand behind the victim and put both your arms around the upper part of the abdomen.
  - Make sure the victim is bending well forwards so that when the obstructing object is dislodged it comes out of the mouth rather than goes further down the airway.
  - Clench your fist and place it between the umbilicus (navel) and xiphisternum (bottom tip of the sternum). Grasp it with your other hand.
  - Pull sharply inwards and upwards; the obstructing object should be dislodged.
  - If the obstruction is still not relieved, recheck the mouth for any obstruction that can be reached with a finger, and continue alternating five back blows with five abdominal thrusts.
4. If the victim at any time becomes unconscious, this may result in the relaxation of the muscles around the larynx (voice box) and allow air to pass down into the lungs. If at any time the choking victim loses consciousness, carry out the following sequence of life support:
- Tilt the victim's head and remove any visible obstruction from the mouth.
- Open their airway further by lifting their chin.

- Check for breathing by looking, listening, and feeling.
- Attempt to give two effective rescue breaths.
- If effective breaths can be achieved within five attempts:
  - Check for signs of a circulation.
  - Start chest compressions and/or rescue breaths as appropriate.
- If effective breaths cannot be achieved within five attempts:
  - Start chest compressions immediately to relieve the obstruction. Do not check for signs of a circulation.
  - After 15 compressions, check the mouth for any obstruction, then attempt further rescue breaths.
  - Continue to give cycles of 15 compressions followed by attempts at rescue breaths.
- If at any time effective breaths can be achieved:
  - Check for signs of a circulation.
  - Continue chest compressions and/or rescue breaths as appropriate.

Long-term management
If the blockage is stubborn and cannot be dislodged, hospital transfer should be instituted without delay.

Chapter 7

Drug-related emergencies

Introduction

This chapter will briefly cover the following drug-related emergencies:
- Overdose—including the possibility of drug interactions
- Allergy
- Idiosyncratic reactions.

Drug reactions can be classified into a number of groups, each of which warrant a textbook of their own. Drugs may cause:
- Side-effects: common non-therapeutic responses to drugs (e.g. gastro-intestinal upset to non-steroidal anti-inflammatory drugs)
- Toxic effects: usually from overdose and have widely varying presentations
- Allergic reactions: a range of responses in patients sensitized to a drug
- Drug interactions
- Idiosyncratic reactions.

Drug-related emergencies are a significant cause of morbidity.

Overdose

Excess of any drug can cause adverse effects. It is pharmacology at its simplest: more drug = more effect. The most common risk of overdose in dentistry is with local anaesthetics, particularly in small children.

Diagnosis

- Excitement
- Anxiety
- Confusion
- Hypotension
- Loss of consciousness and collapse.

Exclusions

- Faint
- Hypoglycaemia
- Other causes of collapse.

Immediate action

- Stop treatment
- Reassure patient
- Lie patient back.

Follow-up action

- Seek help
- Monitor pulse manually or with oximeter
- Oxygen via face mask
- Check blood sugar if possible
- If very prolonged, refer to emergency services.

Risk factors

- Extremes of age
- Four-quadrant dentistry
- Intravascular injections.

Diagnosis in the dental surgery

Diagnosis will depend on the presenting signs and symptoms. The typical presentation is as outlined above. Overdose with local anaesthetic is completely avoidable if adequate risk assessment is carried out and maximum doses are not exceeded.

Other drug overdoses are rare in the dental surgery. Very occasionally, a patient may present having taken too much analgesia over a number of days. Advice should be sought from the *British National Formulary* (*BNF*) and from your local Emergency Department. If in any doubt, a referral to hospital is appropriate.

Overdose of drugs may be actual (too much drug is given) or relative (where high blood levels are achieved by a normal dose). In the case of local anaesthetic agents, it is possible to reach toxic blood levels by intravenous injection (especially in children). An important preventive measure in this case is careful aspiration prior to injection of local anaesthetic agents.

Drug interactions

It is very important to consider drug interactions in any discussion of overdose. There are two main types of drug interaction:

- Pharmacodynamic
- Pharmacokinetic.

Pharmacodynamic interactions

These occur between drugs with similar clinical effects or side-effects. They are usually predictable given a basic knowledge of pharmacology and appear in most, if not all, patients.

Sometimes the effects are merely an additive effect, where the effect of the combination is equivalent to the sum of the individual components (i.e. the effect of drugs a and b is equivalent to the sum of the effects of drug a and the effects of drug b given separately).

It is possible that drugs can have a synergistic effect. In this case, the effect of the combination is greater than the effect of the sum of the separate effects. In some cases, this can be quite pronounced with a three- to four-fold increase in predicated effects (and side-effects).

Pharmacokinetic interactions

These occur when one drug affects the absorption, distribution, metabolism, or excretion of another. They are not easily predicted and affect only a small proportion of users. The drugs that interact in this way are different in their clinical effects and the interaction is not predictable from a basic knowledge of pharmacology. The only way to prevent such interactions between drugs that the patient is taking and those administered by the dentist is to check the drug history against a reference document.

Appendix 1 of the *BNF*, an indispensable guide on all aspects of prescribing for the practising dentist, is devoted in its entirety to drug interactions. The *BNF* describes many known drug interactions but marks a category it calls 'Hazardous interactions' in bold and describes these as potentially hazardous. These are the interactions that the dental team should be particularly aware of and avoid.

Risk assessment

With an aging population seeking more complicated care and comorbidities becoming more common, it is vital that, in assessing the risk for any individual patient, their full drug history is taken into account. Many patients are poor at recalling the drugs they are prescribed. Patients who cannot recall their drug history should be asked to bring a list of medication or a repeat prescription form for the dental team's information.

Management

Drug interactions are a group of conditions that should be avoided, rather than managed once they occur.

Drug interactions are very common and there is extensive information about known drug interaction in the *BNF*. Dentists should be familiar with how to access this information and do so regularly. All healthcare professionals should have a low threshold of suspicion if a patient reacts in an unexpected way to a drug. All such reactions should be reported using the Committee on Safety of Medicine yellow cards.

Drug allergy

Allergy may occur to many of the drugs used in dentistry including the penicillin group of antibiotics and, rarely, to local anaesthetic. Presentation can vary widely from mild swelling to full-blown anaphylactic shock (see Chapter 3).

Diagnosis

- Presentation varies widely
- Erythema of face
- Itching
- Oedema
- Wheeze
- Loss of consciousness
- Pulse weak and rapid
- Blood pressure low and may be difficult to record.

Exclusions

- Idiosyncratic reaction
- Other causes of collapse.

Immediate management

- Stop treatment
- Talk to patient
- Lie patient flat with legs raised
- Administer high-flow oxygen via face mask
- Seek help if no improvement.

Delayed management

- 0.5–1mg adrenaline intramuscularly
- Monitor clinically and electronically if possible
- Repeat adrenaline every 60 seconds if no or limited response
- Arrange hospital admission
- Continued adrenaline
- Antihistamine and steroid treatment
- Intravenous fluids
- Possible intubation.

Risk factors

- Atopic individuals—asthma, eczema, hay fever
- Contact with common allergens—latex, penicillins.

Diagnosis in the dental surgery

Allergy is part of a continuum from simple angioedema, such as lip swelling, through self-limiting anaphylactic reactions characterized by some of the above symptoms. Patients may have erythema and swelling but no wheeze, for example.

The management of an allergic reaction is the same regardless of the allergen that has provoked the response. As it is no longer recommended that antihistamines and steroids are part of the dental emergency drug box, patients who require pharmacological management of the allergic reaction will require the attention of the emergency medical services.

Idiosyncratic reactions

Idiosyncratic reactions are unexpected or paradoxical reactions to a drug (e.g. a sedative producing excitation).

Diagnosis
- Presentation varies widely
- Unexpected effect following drug administration.

Exclusions
- Overdose reaction
- Allergic reaction
- Hysterical reaction
- Other causes of collapse.

Immediate management
- Stop treatment
- Talk to patient
- Apply symptomatic treatment
- Apply principles of basic life support (see Chapter 9)
- Seek help if no improvement.

Delayed management
- Depends on severity and duration of symptoms
- If in doubt, contact emergency medical services
- Arrange further investigation to reach definitive diagnosis.

Diagnosis in the dental surgery
This type of reaction to medication is, by its very nature, unpredictable both in terms of occurrence and presentation. The diagnosis depends on the observation of a clinical picture that cannot be otherwise explained.

Any idiosyncratic drug reaction should be taken seriously.

Immediate management
The immediate management depends on the application of the principles of basic life support as described in Chapter 9.

The patient should be managed in a position in which they are comfortable, if conscious, or head down with the feet raised if unconscious. The unconscious patient should be maintained with the airway open. Adequate ventilation and circulation should be provided if required (see Chapter 9).

Summary

Summary

It is difficult to be definitive in a short textbook about the wide variation in presentation of drug-related emergencies. It is important to prevent avoidable drug-related emergencies including overdose and known drug interactions.

Those who administer any drug to patients should be aware of the therapeutic effects, side-effects, and drug interactions of the agents they use. The potential toxicity of a drug rests in the hands of the user. Application of the knowledge of the properties of each drug administered will prevent the occurrence of avoidable drug-related emergencies

It is difficult to guarantee to avoid allergic reactions as, by their nature, a patient has to be exposed to a substance before subsequently developing the allergy. The initial exposure (and sometimes many subsequent exposures) will be without adverse effect. The first allergic response will thus be unexpected. Any suspected allergic reactions must be noted in the patient's clinical notes. It is, however, important that the word 'allergy' is not used without an accurate diagnosis. Many patients who have been given intravascular injections of local anaesthetic agent have received the false diagnosis of allergy, and have thus been prevented from benefitting from this valuable therapeutic agent. If the aetiology of the reaction is uncertain, patients should be referred for investigation to a clinical pharmacologist or dermatology department.

Chapter 8

Cardiovascular system-related emergencies

Introduction

This chapter will cover the cardiac causes of emergencies. As such, it will deal with conditions that affect the way blood is pumped around the body. The conditions which are covered affect the efficiency of cardiac function.

Problems with circulation are covered in Chapter 3. The conditions described in Chapter 3 may interrelate with those described here. Unlike the conditions described in this chapter, those in Chapter 3 are primarily related to the functioning of the blood vessels and the ability of the vascular system to effectively channel the cardiac output to the tissues needing perfusion and then return the venous blood to the heart.

The conditions covered in this chapter are:
- Angina
- Myocardial infarction
- Cardiac arrest
- Bradycardia
- Tachycardia.

It is assumed that dental practices will not have either access to or the ability to interpret electrocardiogram (ECG) traces, and thus their diagnosis will not be included.

Management will depend on the use of the drugs and equipment outlined in Chapter 1.

Angina (angina pectoris)

Diagnosis
- Central crushing chest pain
- May radiate to left arm and left side of the mandible
- Pain abates within five minutes of cessation of initiating stimulus or administration of glyceryl trinitrate
- Pulse remains regular throughout period of monitoring.

Exclusions
- Myocardial infarction
- Indigestion.

Immediate management
- Stop dental treatment
- Position patient comfortably
- Administer glyceryl trinitrate
- Administer oxygen.

Follow-up action
- Monitor for resolution of symptoms which should resolve within five minutes
- If known to suffer from angina pectoris, compare with 'normal' attacks
- If abnormal for patient, consider referral for exclusion of myocardial infarction.

Risk factors
- History of ischaemic heart disease, with regular predictable episodes of chest pain
- Patient who is anxious about dental treatment
- Patient with other risk factors for ischaemic heart disease (e.g. obesity or hypertension).

Diagnosis in the dental surgery

Diagnosis in the dental surgery depends on clinical signs and symptoms. The typical presentation is of a central crushing chest pain. The symptoms are often equated with the feeling of a weight on the patient's chest. Medical textbooks quote phrases such as 'like an elephant standing on my chest'.

Pain may be alleviated by sitting the patient up. It may radiate to left side of mandible or down the left arm. It is possible for patients only to have pain in either the left arm or the left side of mandible.

Pain is usually self-limiting once the stress factor has been removed or the patient has had glyceryl trinitrate (a coronary vasodilator) administered. If it lasts for more than 30 minutes it should be regarded as indicative of a myocardial infarction until proved otherwise.

The patient's pulse will be regular.

For many patients, the pain of angina pectoris is a regular occurrence. If the pain is similar to that which is usually experienced, it is likely to be related to similar pathology. Chest pain in a patient who has not experienced it before should be regarded as sinister until proved otherwise.

Exclusions

The two other conditions likely to be confused with angina pectoris are:

- Myocardial infarction
- Indigestion (heart burn).

Myocardial infarction

Myocardial infaction should be suspected when the pain is not self-limiting (of less than 30 minutes' duration), is relieved by the administration of glyceryl tinitrate, is atypical of the patient's normal symptoms, or when the patient's pulse is irregular.

If the practitioner is in any doubt, the patient should be considered as having suffered a myocardial infarction until proved otherwise.

Indigestion (heartburn)

This again presents as a central chest pain, which may be confused with pain of cardiac origin. The patient's history can again be a useful guide, although confusion between cardiac and indigestion pain is amongst the most common medical misdiagnoses.

The pain of GI tract origin will be alleviated by antacids (which the patient may commonly carry). Some patients with heartburn may have the desire to eat, and eating may alleviate symptoms. Patients with angina do not wish to eat.

Despite the possibility of appearing foolish, if in doubt, the pain must be viewed as being of cardiac origin until proved otherwise.

Immediate management

- Assess the patient's level of consciousness
- Airway, breathing, circulation (ABC)
- Monitor and reassure the patient
- If the patient is prescribed glyceryl trinitrate (GTN) and has their medication with them, ask the patient to self-medicate
- Give the patient oxygen via a Hudson mask
- Position the patient as they are most comfortable. Most patients will elect to sit up. This reduces the workload on the myocardium.

Myocardial infarction (MI)

Diagnosis
- Central crushing chest pain of more than 20 minutes' duration
- Pain atypical of patient's normal angina pain
- Irregular pulse.

Exclusions
- Angina pectoris
- Indigestion.

Immediate management
- Stop dental treatment
- Assess consciousness
- ABC
- Analgesia
- Oxygen
- GTN
- Aspirin
- Monitor for cardiac arrest.

Follow-up action
Hospital admission.

Risk factors
- Previous ischaemic heart disease
- Previous myocardial infarction (especially if within the previous three months)
- Diabetes mellitus (myocardial infarction may present without chest pain)
- Obesity
- Hypertension.

Diagnosis in the dental surgery
Unexplained chest pain should be considered as an MI until this has been excluded. (MI is the major cause of death in middle age.)
- Definitive diagnosis in the dental surgery is impossible as it depends on the recording of a 12-lead ECG and the presence of raised cardiac enzyme levels in the blood
- Central crushing chest pain
- May radiate to left side of mandible or left arm
- Pain of more than 20 minutes' duration
- Pain that is atypical in duration or severity from the patient's previous experience of angina
- Irregular pulse.

Exclusions
- Angina attack:
  - pain like patient's usual symptoms
  - pain of limited (less than five minutes') duration
  - pain relieved by administration of GTN.

- Indigestion:
  - burning pain
  - pain that patient equates with normal symptoms of indigestion
  - pain relieved by eating.

Immediate management

- Stop dental treatment
- Position the patient as most comfortable. Normally, patients will want to sit up as this reduces venous return and, thus, the workload on the myocardium
- Assess consciousness. Monitor the patient's state of consciousness and reassure them. Patients often feel a sense of impending doom
- ABC. Ensure that the airway, breathing, and circulation are adequate for the maintenance of cerebral function.
- Analgesia. The pain of myocardial infarction can be severe. The stress that this causes will increase the workload on the myocardium. The most effective and available analgesic in the dental environment is nitrous oxide.
- Oxygen should be administered. If nitrous oxide is administered as an analgesic, then supplementary oxygen will be given concurrently.
- GTN
- Aspirin. This will help to dissolve any thrombus that is occluding the coronary artery
- Monitor for cardiac arrest. MI is the most common cause of cardiac arrest, and the patient's level of consciousness and pulse should be regularly monitored.

Subsequent management

All patients who have suffered a suspected MI in the dental environment should be sent by ambulance to hospital. If in doubt, hospital admission should be arranged. Despite the potential for appearing foolish, it is better to send a patient who has not suffered an MI to hospital than to send a patient who has suffered an MI home.

Other considerations

MI in the dental environment is rare but should not be undiagnosed. Patients who have diabetes mellitus can have a 'silent MI' (i.e. MI without chest pain). The patient will have other symptoms such as:

- Breathlessness
- Sense of impending doom
- General feeling of weakness and being unwell.

Cardiac arrest

Diagnosis
Patient is unconscious and has no pulse.

Exclusions
- Faint
- Epileptic fit
- MI
- Drug overdose.

Immediate management
- Stop any dental treatment
- Assess level of consciousness
- ABC
- Call for paramedic ambulance
- Continue cardiopulmonary resuscitation (CPR) until help arrives.

Follow-up action
When successfully resuscitated, the patient must be evacuated to hospital.

Risk factors
- Previous ischaemic heart disease
- Recent MI.

Diagnosis in the dental surgery

The clinical diagnosis of cardiac arrest depends on the patient being unconscious (i.e. does not respond to shake and shout) and having no palpable carotid pulse.

Further diagnosis as to the type of cardiac arrest depends on an ECG diagnosis. This will be discussed in Chapter 10.

Exclusions

All other causes of unconsciousness must be excluded. By definition, if a pulse is present, the patient has not suffered a cardiac arrest.

Immediate management

Survival depends on early basic life support (see Chapter 9) and early access to advanced life support (see Chapter 10).
- Stop any dental treatment
- Assess level of consciousness
- Assess ABC
- Once cardiac arrest is confirmed, call for a paramedic ambulance
- Commence CPR
- Continue CPR until help arrives
- Assist paramedic team in management of the patient.

Subsequent management

- The subsequent management will depend on the type of cardiac arrest (see Chapter 10)
- In adults, the most likely cause is ventricular fibrillation. This will be treated by defibrillation
- The algorithms for the management of the different types of cardiac arrest are given in Chapter 10.

Paediatric considerations

- In children, the primary cause of cardiac arrest is usually respiratory
- In the paediatric patient, two rescue breaths are given to the patient prior to any other stage in the 'chain of survival' (see Chapters 9 and 10).

Bradycardia

Diagnosis
* Patient has a slow heart rate of less than 60 beats per minute

or

* Patient's heart rate is too slow to maintain haemodynamic stability.

(NB The rate must be significantly lower than normal for the patient. It is worth noting that some athletes have a resting heart rate well below 60 and that this is normal for them.)

Immediate action
* Stop any dental treatment
* Assess level of consciousness
* ABC
* Give oxygen
* Assess for adverse signs of bradycardia:
  * systolic blood pressure <90mmHg
  * heart rate <40 beats per minute
  * signs of heart failure
  * irregular pulse.
* Call emergency services—urgency greatest if adverse signs present
* Monitor for deterioration.

Diagnosis in the dental surgery

The diagnosis will be a clinical diagnosis on the basis of an observed change in heart rate. An accurate diagnosis is impossible without an ECG and, thus, early access to this is the main aim of management.

Exclusions

Abnormally slow pulse rate that is normal for the patient.

Immediate management

The management in the dental environment is limited by the fact that the diagnosis will be a clinical diagnosis only. The patient should be monitored, reassured, and evacuated for definitive treatment as soon as possible.

Subsequent management

The subsequent management will depend on the severity and cause of the bardycardia. It may include pharmacological treatment using atropine or epinephrine or pacing of the myocardium via external or internal pacers. This is beyond the scope of management in the dental setting.

Tachycardia

Diagnosis
Patient has an unacceptably fast pulse (>150 beats per minute).

Immediate management
- Stop any dental treatment
- Assess level of consciousness
- ABC
- Administer oxygen
- Assess for adverse signs of tachycardia:
  - systolic blood pressure less than 90mmHg
  - heart rate >150 beats per minute
  - chest pain
  - heart failure
- Call emergency services—urgency greatest if adverse signs present
- Monitor for deterioration.

Diagnosis in the dental surgery

The diagnosis is based on a clinical diagnosis of a fast pulse. The only other assessment that is possible is the presence or absence of adverse signs.

Exclusions

- Intravascular injection of epinephrine containing local anaesthetic
- Anaphylactic reaction.

Immediate management

- There is little other than reassurance and monitoring that can be done for these patients in the dental environment.
- Any dental treatment should be stopped and the patient positioned as they are most comfortable
- The patient should be assessed as for all emergencies:
  - level of consciousness
  - ABC
- Oxygen should be administered to aid the myocardium's increased demand as a result of the tachycardia
- The emergency services should be called to arrange the transfer of the patient to hospital
- The patient must be carefully monitored.

Subsequent management

Subsequent management will depend on the severity and cause of the tachycardia. It may include:
- Pharmacological treatment with adenosine or amiodarone
- Cardioversion of the myocardium.

Cardioversion is similar to defibrillation but involves the delivery of a smaller charge synchronized to the period of ventricular depolarization. This is beyond the scope of management in the dental setting.

Summary

The majority of the conditions described in this chapter will require hospital intervention. There is the potential for the progression of these conditions to more serious, potentially fatal sequellae such as cardiac arrest. There is, however, usually the opportunity to arrange the appropriate transfer for further help. An appreciation of the condition that the patient is suffering allows appropriate initial treatment. It is also important to appear calm and confident during the management of these conditions. If the patient becomes agitated or stressed, the likelihood of serious sequellae increases. Effective communication and a confident air are the best way of reducing the patient's stress.

Basic life support

Introduction

Aim

The aim of basic life support (BLS) is to maintain adequate ventilation and circulation until treatment to reverse the underlying cause of cardiorespiratory arrest can be undertaken.

Importance of prompt institution of BLS

Delays in starting BLS significantly reduce the likelihood of a successful outcome. Failure to adequately perfuse the brain with oxygenated blood for 3–4 minutes will result in irreversible cerebral damage.

The only permissible delay in commencing BLS is the time taken to summon help in the form of a cardiac arrest team or paramedic ambulance.

Concept of BLS

BLS is the maintenance of effective ventilation and circulation without the use of any equipment. This is how BLS would be expected to be delivered by lay rescuers. Within the dental environment, it is anticipated that the airway adjuncts that were discussed in Chapter 1 will be available. The reader may be unfortunate enough to encounter a cardiac arrest away from their workplace, and thus BLS without adjuncts is discussed. The sequence described here is for the management of cardiac arrest, not for the management of victims of trauma. Modifications for the trauma scenario will be considered in a separate section.

History of BLS

Although cardiac compressions were originally described in the late nineteenth century, BLS as we understand it today was introduced in 1960. Effective BLS is one of the few interventions proved to have a positive effect on the outcome of a cardiac arrest.

Sequence of BLS for healthcare personnel where trauma to the cervical spine is not suspected

The sequence can be summarized as:
- Ensure it is safe to approach.
- Assess victim's level of consciousness.
- Shout for help.
- A—assess airway
- B—assess breathing

1. Ensure that it is safe to approach the victim.
2. Assess whether the victim is conscious—gently grasp the victim's shoulders and, in a loud voice, ask 'Are you all right?' (Fig. 9.1).
3. If victim responds to stimulus—response may be verbal or by moving/groaning:
   - Do not move the victim (unless it is dangerous to leave him/her where found).
   - Monitor the victim's condition regularly to assess for improvement or deterioration.
   - Get further assistance if required.
4. If no response from victim:
   - Shout for help.
   - If necessary for assessment, move victim onto his/her back.
   - Open the airway. Tilt the victim's head back by placing a hand on the forehead. The hand position should allow the thumb and forefinger to be used to close the nostrils should exhaled air respiration (EAR) be required.
   - With the victim's mouth open, look for obstructions (Fig. 9.2). Any visible obstruction should be removed. Dentures, if well fitting, should be left *in situ* to support the contour of the face. Loose dentures should be removed. If there is no obvious obstruction, blind finger sweeps and use of suction should be avoided lest an unseen obstruction is pushed further into the airway or vomiting is induced.

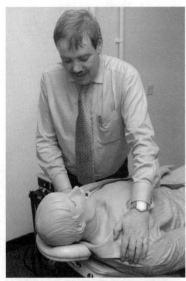

Fig. 9.1 'Shake and shout' to establish level of consciousness.

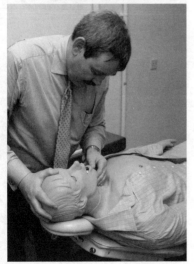

Fig. 9.2 Assessment of the airway for obvious signs of obstruction.

- Keeping the airway open, look, listen, and feel for signs of breathing.
  —The rescuer should position themselves so they can see any attempted chest movements, and listen for sounds of breathing. Positioning their cheek just over the patient allows the rescuer to feel the movement of air.
  —This process should take up to 10 seconds. If no effective breaths are felt in 10 seconds, cardiorespiratory arrest is diagnosed.
5. If victim is breathing normally:
  - Turn the victim into the recovery position (Fig. 9.3).
  - Monitor regularly for change in the victim's condition.
  - Summon assistance by either sending someone or, if alone, it may mean leaving the victim.
6. If victim is not making any effective ventilatory efforts—there are either no signs of breathing or occasional weak gasps:
  - Summon assistance, if necessary leaving the victim.
  - Commence chest compressions (see 'Sequence of chest compressions').
  - Compressions and ventilations continue at a ratio of 30:2. This ratio is maintained regardless of the number of rescuers.
  - Cardiopulmonary resuscitation (CPR) is maintained until:
    —Help arrives to relieve the rescuer(s).
    —The rescuer(s) become exhausted.
    —The victim shows signs of life. This is always included as an indication to cease CPR despite the recognition that CPR will not reverse a cardiac arrest. It is included here for completeness.

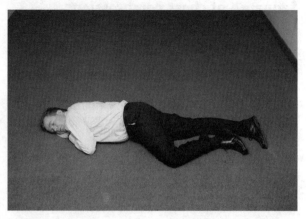

Fig. 9.3 The recovery position.

Sequence of chest compressions (Fig. 9.4)

1. Place the heel of one hand in the middle of the sternum.
2. Place the heel of the other hand on top of the hand which is on the sternum.
3. Extend your fingers so that they are not in contact with the victim's ribs (many people prefer to interlock their fingers).
4. Position your shoulders vertically above the victim's sternum.
5. Keeping elbows straight, press down to compress the sternum 4–5cm (1.5–2").
6. Release the pressure without losing contact with the chest wall.
7. Allow the chest to recoil to its resting position.
8. Repeat compressions at a rate of approximately 100 per minute.
   - The correct rate is achieved by counting '1 - and - 2 - and - 3 - and - 4' etc.
   - The time for compression and recoil should be the same.
9. After 30 compressions, give two effective inflations of the lungs.
   - The airway will have to be reopened with head tilt and chin lift.
10. Return hands to the correct position and continue.

Notes on chest compressions

- The aim is to compress the chest by about a third of its depth. For an adult, this will be approximately 4–5cm (1.5–2").
- The pressure must be applied to the middle of the sternum.
- Pressure must not be applied to the abdomen or the tip of the sternum.
- Pressure must not be applied to the ribs.
- Pressure must be applied vertically in a firm but controlled fashion.
- Erratic or violent forces should be avoided as they could cause harm.
- The compression and recoil phase should take about the same amount of time.
- The sequence of BLS should only be interrupted for advanced life support (ALS) procedures.
- BLS should only be stopped to check for a pulse if the victim appears to respond (very unlikely) or to check the success of ALS procedures (see Chapter 10).

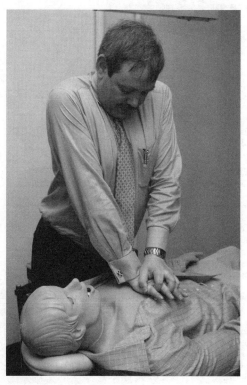

Fig. 9.4 Chest compressions.

Sequence of EAR (Fig. 9.5)

1. Ensure adequate head tilt and chin lift to open the airway.
2. Pinch the nostrils closed with the thumb and index finger of the hand that is on the victim's forehead.
3. Maintaining chin lift, open the mouth a little.
4. Take a moderate breath.
5. Place lips over the victim's mouth ensuring an airtight seal.
6. Blow steadily into victim's mouth. (Take no longer than one second.)
7. Watch for the chest rise. (Do not inflate the chest to more than a normal breath.)
8. Maintaining head tilt and chin lift, remove mouth from the victim's and turn head to watch the chest fall.
9. Repeat.

Notes on EAR

- There should be no great resistance to inflation of the victim's lungs
- Each rescue breath should only take about one second
- Avoid over inflating the lungs or using excessive force. This will inflate the stomach and may lead to regurgitation
- Each inflation should make the chest rise the equivalent of a 'normal' breath (for the patient)
- The chest should return to the rest position between ventilations. This may take between two and four seconds
- A rescue breath may thus take up to five seconds for both inflation and exhalation.
- It is more important that the chest is allowed to fall to complete exhalation than that the ventilations are given at the rate of 10 per minute
- If difficulties are encountered during attempted EAR, the victim's mouth should be rechecked for obstructions. The position of the head can be adjusted to increase the opening of the airway
- Only have two attempts to provide EAR between each set of compressions.

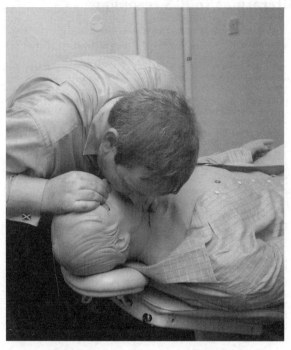

Fig. 9.5 Exhaled air restoration.

Alterations to BLS technique: two-person CPR

A single rescuer can use the technique described above. However, it is more efficient to have two rescuers. In two-person CPR, one carries out the ventilations and the other the compressions. This is more efficient as there is less time lost in changing from ventilations to compressions and back.

When two rescuers are present, one can commence CPR while the other goes to summon help. Two-person CPR can be started on their return.

Notes on two-person CPR

- If one rescuer sends another to summon help, always tell them to return.
- It is easier if the two rescuers work from opposite sides of the victim.
- If one rescuer is less trained than the other, it is easier to ask them to perform chest compressions.
- The ratio of compressions to ventilations remains 30:2.
- A minimum of delay between compressions is achieved if the rescuer providing compressions counts as described above.
- During ventilations, the rescuer providing compressions does not remove their hands from the victim's chest. It is important not to apply pressure, but to allow the chest to rise.
- Head tilt/chin lift is maintained at all times.
- Compressions cease to allow ventilations, but resume immediately after the second ventilation (allowing the rescuer to remove their lips from contact with the victim's face).
- Providing compressions is significantly more tiring than providing ventilations. Rescuers should plan to swap roles if required. This should be accomplished with as little disruption to CPR as possible.

Alternative methods of ventilation

Although there is little evidence of untoward effects of mouth-to-mouth ventilation for the rescuer, many are unwilling to perform this on unknown victims of cardiac arrest.

Mouth-to-nose ventilation

Mouth-to-nose ventilation may be used in preference to mouth-to-mouth ventilation in edentulous patients without dentures or where loose dentures have had to be removed and an effective seal cannot be made. It may also be preferable if a patient has collapsed during or immediately after intra-oral surgery and there is a significant amount of blood in the victim's mouth.

Mouth-to-mask ventilation

A number of devices are available that place a barrier between the rescuer and victim. The use of such devices makes EAR more acceptable to the rescuer, who does not have to come into such intimate contact with the victim.

The pocket mask (Fig. 9.6) is based on a clear anaesthetic mask with a one-way valve added. The mask is clear so that condensation from the air exhaled by the victim can be seen. It will also allow any blood or vomit that might be present to be seen.

Some of the devices also have a port that enables supplementary oxygen to be added increasing the given concentration from the 16% contained in expired air to approximately 40%. In the case of a mask that does not have a port for oxygen to be added, the tube from the oxygen cylinder can be placed under the edge of the mask. The oxygen should be set at a flow rate of 10–15 litres per minute. The use of supplemental oxygen will not provide ventilation unless mouth-to-mask ventilation is used to propel the oxygen into the victim's lungs.

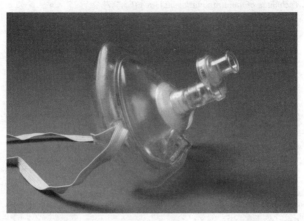

Fig. 9.6 The pocket mask with one-way valve.

Technique of mouth-to-mask ventilation (Fig. 9.7)
1. Mouth-to-mask ventilation is best achieved from behind the patient.
2. The mask is placed over the mouth and nose (with the point towards the nose).
3. The thumbs of both hands hold the mask in place while the fingers lift the lower border of the mandible to open the airway.
4. Air is blown through the valve to inflate the lungs.
5. The chest should be seen to rise.
6. When the inflation ceases, the chest should be seen to fall.

Notes on mouth-to mask ventilation
- The mask has to be pressed tightly onto the victim's face to produce an airtight seal.
- Any leaks around the mask should be eliminated by altering the position of the hands and/or increasing the opening of the airway.
- Using the pocket mask is not a substitute for adequate opening of the airway.
- As with mouth-to-mouth ventilation, the temptation to overinflate the victim's lungs must be resisted to prevent gastric inflation.

Bag-valve-mask ventilation

The use of a bag-valve-mask ventilation system allows the administration of a significantly higher concentration of oxygen than either of the previous two methods of ventilation.

The bag-valve-mask is difficult for a single rescuer to use unless experienced. One hand has to maintain an adequate degree of chin lift while also maintaining an airtight seal between the mask and the face. The other hand has to compress the bag adequately to produce sufficient inflation of the lungs. As a general principle, good mouth-to-mouth ventilation is preferable to poor bag-valve-mask ventilation.

The bag-valve-mask system can be effectively used by two rescuers (Fig. 9.8).
1. The oxygen supply is connected to the port and the reservoir bag allowed to fill.
2. The rescuer who is to maintain the airway kneels behind the victim's head and holds the mask as described for the pocket mask above.
3. The second rescuer positions himself/herself beside the victim and squeezes the bag with both hands. In this case, the rescuer who provides the inflations by squeezing the bag can also carry out chest compressions if required.
- The use of the bag-valve-mask is not a substitute for good opening of the airway or provision of a good seal between the mask and the victim's face.

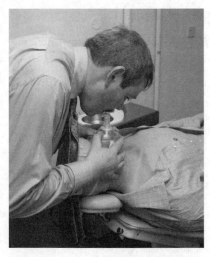

Fig. 9.7 Mouth-to-mask ventilation using the pocket mask.

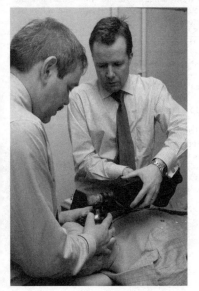

Fig. 9.8 The use of bag-value-mask ventilation by two rescuers.

The use of airway adjuncts: the oropharyngeal airway

The basic technique for opening the airway in an unconscious casualty in the dental environment is the head tilt/chin lift. The use of airway adjuncts can improve the opening of the airway. The most commonly available in the dental environment is the oropharyngeal airway. Other adjuncts will be described in Chapter 10.

The oropharyngeal or Guedel (Fig. 9.9) airway will help to prevent the posterior third of the tongue from blocking the unconscious patient's airway by falling back against the posterior pharyngeal wall. It will not maintain the airway in the absence of head tilt and chin lift, but it can reduce the degree of opening required to keep the airway patent.

Guedel airways are provided in a range of sizes to fit all. The correct size is selected by measuring from the incisor teeth to the angle of the mandible (Fig. 9.10).

Technique for insertion of the Guedel airway
1. The correct size is selected.
2. The airway is opened by head tilt and chin lift.
3. The Guedel airway is inserted upside down (with the convex side facing the tongue).
4. Once the end of the airway reaches the junction of the hard and soft palate, it is rotated through 180° and advanced so that the unflanged end lies behind the posterior third of the tongue.

Notes on placement of the Guedel airway
- Placing the airway initially inverted and then rotating it through 180° minimizes the chances of pushing the tongue back and aggravating the airway obstruction.
- The Guedel airway is not well tolerated unless the victim is deeply unconscious.
- Should the victim start to cough or gag on the airway it should be removed.
- Once correctly inserted, the flange will sit inside the upper lip, anterior to the incisor teeth (or edentulous ridge).
- Correct insertion will be indicated by an improvement in the ease of maintenance of the airway.
- The airway should be assessed by maintaining head tilt and chin lift, then employing the look, listen, and feel technique that was described earlier in this chapter.

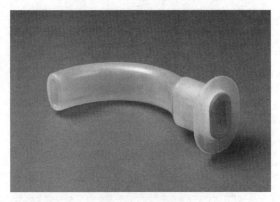

Fig. 9.9 The oropharyngeal airway (Guedel airway).

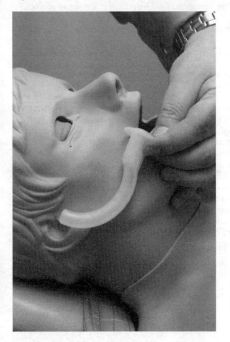

Fig. 9.10 Selection of the correction size of oropharyngeal airway. The correct size extends from the angle of the mouth to the anterior of the ear.

The recovery position

The recovery position is used either for an unconscious casualty who is breathing and has an adequate pulse or for post-resuscitation care when the victim remains unconscious.

The recovery position allows an adequate airway to be maintained and minimizes the risk of aspiration should the victim vomit.

Sequence for placing victim in the recovery position (Fig. 9.11)

Prior to moving the victim, it is important to remove any potential cause of pressure sores. The victim's glasses (if worn) should be removed. Any items such as keys in the victim's pocket should be removed.

1. Kneel beside the victim just to the head side of the hips.
2. Move the arm nearest you perpendicular to the body, with the elbow bent and the palm uppermost.
3. Take hold of the opposite leg and pull/bend the knee, keeping the foot in contact with the ground. (Tucking the toe of the foot under the knee of the leg nearest you will help to keep the leg as you positioned it.)
4. Take hold of the hand opposite and bring the arm across the victim's chest.
5. Place the back of the victim's opposite hand against the cheek nearest you.
6. Use the opposite leg as a lever to roll the victim towards you. (As you roll the victim ensure that you maintain control of the victim's head and neck.)
7. Once lying on his/her side, position the victim's upper leg so that the thigh is at right angles to the body and that the lower leg is at right angles to the thigh.
8. The head should be positioned with the neck extended to ensure that the airway remains open.
9. The hand that is under the cheek can be positioned to maintain an adequate head position.

Once in the recovery position, the victim should be monitored regularly for signs of improvement or deterioration. Checks should be made that the victim continues to breath and has an adequate circulation. The perfusion of the lower arm must also be checked regularly.

Should the victim need to remain in the recovery position for longer than 30 minutes, they should be turned onto the opposite side.

The sequence of placing a patient in the recovery position:

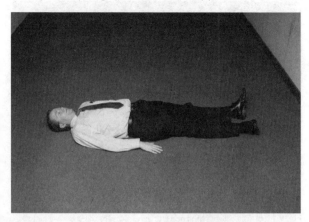

Fig. 9.11(a) An unconscious patient lying on their back. This patient may have an obstructed airway.

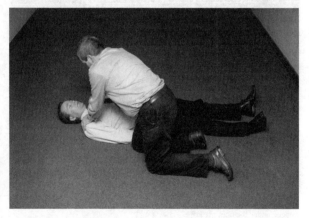

Fig. 9.11(b) The patient should be assessed. The unconscious patient who is breathing and has a circulation is best protected in the recovery position.

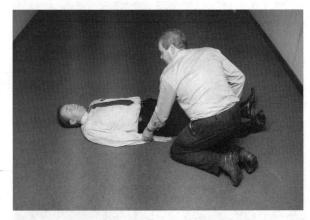

Fig. 9.11(c) The patient's hand nearest the rescuer is placed under the buttock.

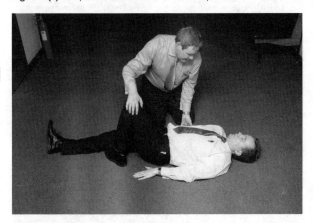

Fig. 9.11(d) The patient's leg opposite the rescuer is raised so that the foot is wedged under the opposite knee.

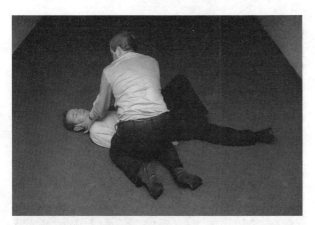

Fig. 9.11(e) The patient's opposite arm is moved so that the back of the hand is against the cheek nearest the rescuer.

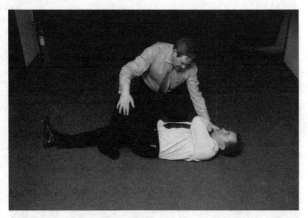

Fig. 9.11(f) The patient is then turned towards the rescuer. The patient's head and neck are supported during this process

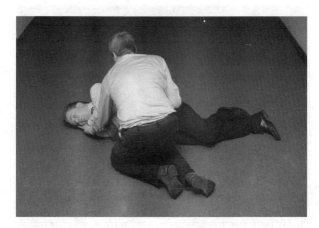

Fig. 9.11(g) The patient is then turned towards the rescuer. The patient's head and neck are supported during this process

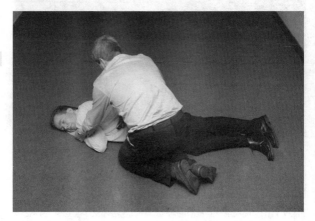

Fig. 9.11(h) The patient's airway is extended to ensure it stays open.

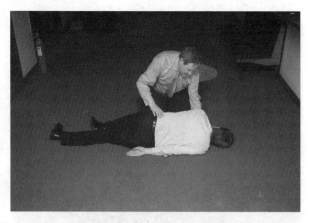

Fig. 9.11(i) The patient's lower arm is brought just behind them and the upper knee is brought forward to prevent the patient rolling onto either their front or back.

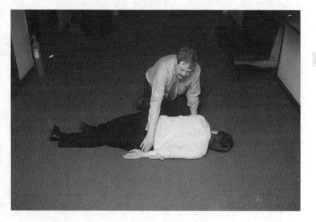

Fig. 9.11(j) The radial pulse in the patient's lower arm is checked to confirm that there is adequate perfusion of the limb.

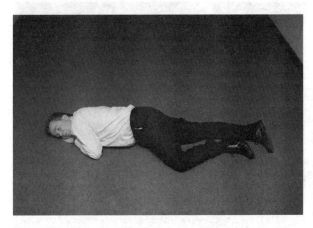

Fig. 9.11(k) In this position, the patient's airway remains patent. The patient should continue to be monitored until the return of consciousness or medical assistance arrives.

Modifications to BLS for the paediatric patient

Paediatric patients can be divided into children and infants:
- A child is considered to be between one and eight years.
- An infant is considered to be under one year.

The principles of BLS in paediatric patients are the same as in adults—namely, that cerebral oxygenation is maintained.

Definitions
- Paediatric BLS applies to those under the age of puberty.
- An infant is defined as a child of less than one year of age.
- A child is defined as being between the ages of one year and puberty.

The sequence of actions
The sequence of actions in paediatric BLS recognizes that cardiac arrest is almost always secondary to respiratory events:
1. Ensure there is no further danger to the child or the rescuer.
2. Assess responsiveness:
   - Shake and shout:
     —If responds, do not move unless in danger.
     —If no response, shout for help then assess Airway, Breathing, and Circulation (if confident that it can be accurately assessed in less than 10 seconds). If breathing absent or infrequent and irregular, then give 5 rescue breaths.

EAR in the child
EAR in the child is essentially the same as EAR for those over the age of puberty. The volume of air blown into the child's lungs must be sufficient to cause the chest to rise, but will be less than required for an adult patient.

EAR in the infant
The principles are the same for infants as for children. Due to the small size of the infant's face, it is frequently easier to use mouth to mouth-and-nose ventilation. In this case, the rescuer's mouth forms a seal over the victim's mouth and nose.

In larger infants, the mouth-to-nose method of EAR may be used when it is difficult to provide an adequate seal over both mouth and nose.

In infants, overextension of the neck can cause respiratory obstruction and, thus, repositioning the infant's head and neck in a more neutral position may improve ventilation.

Assessing circulation in paediatric patients
- In children, circulation is assessed by checking the carotid pulse, as in adults.
- In infants, circulation is assessed by checking the brachial pulse on the inner aspect of the upper arm.
- This process should only be undertaken by those trained in assessing the pulse and must take no longer than 10 seconds.

Infants and children have a higher pulse rate than adults. Thus, in those under eight years, a pulse rate of under 60 per minute is considered as equivalent to a status of cardiac arrest.

Chest compressions for infants

For a single rescuer

1. Once the sternum has been located, the tips of two fingers are placed one finger's width above where the lowest ribs join in the middle.
2. The sternum is depressed by approximately one third of the depth of the chest.
3. This is repeated at a rate of 100 compressions per minute.
4. After 15 compressions, two effective rescue breaths are given.
5. The resuscitation is continued at a ratio of 15:2, although the lone rescuer may use a ratio of 30:2, particularly if having difficulty with the transition between compressions and ventilations.

For more than one rescuer

1. Place thumbs over the lower half of the sternum as described above.
2. The fingers encircle chest, supporting the back.
3. The sternum is compressed to between one third and a half its depth with the thumbs.
4. The ratio and rate are as above.
5. The second rescuer manages the airway and EAR.

Chest compressions for a child

1. The heel of one hand is placed over the lower half of the sternum as above.
2. The fingers are lifted to prevent pressure being applied to the ribs.
3. With the shoulder vertically over the sternum and the arm straight, compress the sternum to approximately one third to a half of the depth of the chest.
4. Release the pressure.
5. Repeat at a rate of 100 per minute.
6. After five compressions, give one effective rescue breath.
7. Continue at a ratio of five compressions to one ventilation.

Chest compressions for larger children

It may be necessary to use the adult technique for larger children.

Summoning assistance

As with adults, it is vital to summon assistance as soon as possible.

When there is more than one rescuer present, one should go for help and then return, while the other starts resuscitation.

A lone rescuer should perform resuscitation for approximately one minute prior to going for help. If the infant or child is small, it may be possible for the rescuer to carry them. The BLS is performed for a minute, as most childhood cardiac arrests are secondary to hypoxia. The one minute of BLS will provide a reservoir of oxygen to limit the deterioration during the process of summoning help.

The only exception to the above is where the victim is known to have heart disease and has collapsed suddenly without a traumatic or toxic cause. In such cases, an arrythmia is the probable cause and early defibrillation is required.

The recovery position is similar for adults and children.

The management of airway obstruction in the paediatric patient

The management of airway obstruction is similar in adults and children.

If the child is attempting to clear the obstruction, his/her own efforts should be encouraged. Intervention should only be considered when these attempts prove to be ineffective or breathing is inadequate.

- Blind finger sweeps should be avoided as these may damage soft tissues or force the obstruction further into the airway.
- As with adults, a sharp increase in intrathoracic pressure is required.

Sequence to clear foreign body obstruction in the child

Effective cough

If the child is coughing effectively, encourage coughing and monitor for relief of obstruction or deterioration to ineffective cough.

Ineffective cough, conscious

1. Perform five back blows (see above).
2. Perform five chest thrusts.
   - Turn child onto back with head lower than chest and airway open.
   - Give up to five chest thrusts. (Chest for infants, abdominal for child >1 year.)
     —Chest thrusts are similar to chest compressions.
     —Chest thrusts should be at a rate of 20 per minute.
     —Chest thrusts should be 'sharper' than chest compressions.
3. Check in mouth to see if obstruction now visible—if so, remove.
4. Open airway and reassess breathing.
5. If child breathing, turn to recovery position and monitor.
6. If child not breathing:
   - Attempt EAR for five breaths.
   - Start CPR.

Sequence to clear foreign body obstruction in the infant

The sequence is essentially the same as for the child but:

- Abdominal thrusts are contraindicated due to the high chance of damaging the internal organs.
- All cycles comprise five back blows and five chest thrusts.

Summary

BLS is a method of reducing the deterioration that the victim will suffer prior to the instigation of immediate or advanced life support. As such, it is an essential link in the chain of survival. Proficiency in BLS is the cornerstone of medical emergency management. The routines described here should be rehearsed by all teams providing dental care so that, in the unlikely event of a medical emergency in the dental environment, the victim will have the greatest chance of survival.

Immediate and advanced life support

Introduction

Immediate (ILS) and advanced life support (ALS) are levels of training defined by the Resuscitation Council. The only dental teams who require to be competent at ILS or ALS are those involved in delivering advanced conscious sedation techniques (such as multiple intravenous drug techniques) or those treating patients under general anaesthesia.

The information in this chapter is aimed at the dentist who is not ILS or ALS trained. Those requiring ILS or ALS training should access courses via the Resuscitation Training Officer at the local hospital. Reading this chapter is not a substitute for attending a course.

The rationale for ILS and ALS

Coronary artery disease is one of the major killers in the twenty-first century. The mean 28-day fatality from acute coronary artery disease episodes is 49% for men and 51% for women. Approximately 33% of those who develop an acute myocardial infarction will die before reaching hospital.

In adults, the most common pattern of electrical activity that is associated with cardiac arrest is a rhythm that can be managed by early defibrillation (ventricular fibrillation or pulseless ventricular tachycardia). The philosophy of ILS and ALS is summed up by the chain of survival. This is illustrated in Fig. 10.1.

Stages in the chain of survival

Early access

If a cardiac arrest occurs outside the hospital setting, immediate access to the emergency medical services is critical to the chances of survival. This is why the first stage of basic life support after confirming cardiac arrest is to call for medical assistance.

Early basic life support (BLS)

BLS, as described in Chapter 9, will decrease the rate of deterioration of the heart and brain. It is thought that in cardiac arrests that occur outside hospital, the early commencement of BLS will dramatically increase the chances of survival.

Early defibrillation

In cardiac arrests that are treatable with defibrillation, the chances of successful defibrillation decrease by about 10% per minute from the onset of cardiac arrest. The debate as to whether defibrillation is part of BLS or ILS/ALS is still ongoing.

Early ALS

If defibrillation successfully restores cardiac output, it is often necessary to institute appropriate post cardiac arrest management to ensure both that the cardiac output is adequate to restore circulation and that the patient does not suffer a further cardiac arrest.

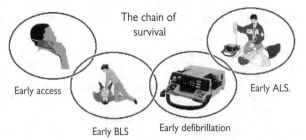

Fig. 10.1 The 'chain of survival'. (Reproduced with permission of Laerdal Medical Ltd., Kent, UK.)

Defibrillation

What is defibrillation?

Defibrillation is a process of resetting the myocardium so that the natural pacemaker can take over and restore the normal electrical and mechanical activity.

In adults, the normal pattern of electrical activity associated with cardiac arrest is ventricular fibrillation. This is produced by a totally disorganized pattern of contraction of the myocardial cells.

Defibrillation involves passing an electrical current across the myocardium to depolarize a critical mass of cardiac muscle. Once the muscle is in the refractory phase, the area of muscle that depolarizes most rapidly will contract first—that is the natural pacemaker (sinoatrial node). Once that occurs, the impulse should spread in the normal pattern.

The electrical charge is delivered across the chest in a direction that will cross the largest mass of heart muscle. This is accomplished by placing the defibrillator paddles or pads in the positions shown in Fig. 10.2.

Although defibrillation has the capacity to be life-saving, electricity is potentially fatal. The most important factor to be considered is safety; it is imperative that no one is in contact with the patient who is being defibrillated. This also includes indirect contact via a medium such as water or fluids.

Use of defibrillators

At one time, defibrillators could only be used by those who were ALS Trained. Traditional defibrillators discharged their charge via paddles held against the patient's chest (Fig. 10.3). The decision as to whether the cardiac rhythm was 'shockable' or not depended on the clinician's interpretation of the electrocardiogram trace.

Recently, automated external defibrillators (AEDs) (Fig. 10.4) have been introduced. These deliver the charge through adhesive pads, and the defibrillator takes the decision as to whether the shock should be delivered. All such defibrillators record the events of cardiac arrests. There has never been an occasion when a shock has been delivered to an inappropriate cardiac rhythm.

Such defibrillators are now widely available. Locations such as railway stations, airports, and some retail outlets have these defibrillators for their clients. The Resuscitation Council has recently indicated that such defibrillators should be available in all locations where healthcare is provided. This would include all areas where dental treatment is provided. The dental regulatory bodies have not yet endorsed such recommendations.

It is the authors' opinion that a requirement for all practices to have an AED is only a matter of time. Although it is difficult to justify in terms of the number of cardiac arrests seen in dental practices, it is more difficult to argue that dental surgeries be exempt from current Resuscitation Council recommendations. How can one rationalize the presence of defibrillators in railway stations etc. but not in environments where healthcare is delivered?

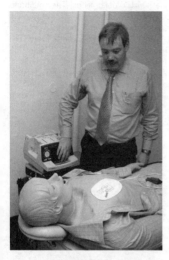

Fig. 10.2 The 'hands free' use of the defibrillator via adhesive pads on the chest.

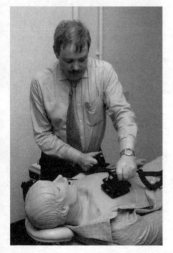

Fig. 10.3 The use of the defibrillator with paddles.

Another recent development is the biphasic defibrillator. The traditional defibrillator passes an electrical current in one direction across the myocardium (monophasic). The biphasic defibrillator passes the current in two directions. This makes the delivery of the charge more efficient. The normal pattern of monophasic charge delivery would be 200 joules followed by a second shock of 200 joules and a third shock of 360 joules. If the cycle has to be repeated, all shocks would be delivered at 360 joules. The normal pattern for a biphasic defibrillator would be to deliver three shocks at a charge of 175 joules. Any further shocks would be at 175 joules.

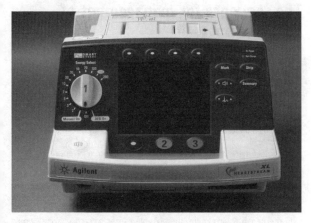

Fig. 10.4 An example of an automated external defibrillator (AED).

The sequence for management of cardiac arrest

The ALS algorithm provides the basis for the management of cardiac arrests. This is reproduced as Fig. 10.5.

Once the ALS team arrives, the algorithm will be followed. This may include endotracheal intubation to secure the patient's airway. The administration of drugs such as epinephrine and amiodorone intravenously is also indicated in patients where a shockable cardiac arrest is present. In patients suffering from a non-shockable cardiac arrest, epinephrine and atropine are indicated. Thus, intravenous access is an integral part of the ALS protocol.

In adults where it has proved impossible to gain intravenous access, it is possible that the drugs can be given via the endotracheal tube. In this case, the dose is doubled. To the uninitiated, the sight of drugs being poured down the tube may appear illogical to the point of being dangerous! Should any member of the dental team see drugs administered in this way, they ought not to be alarmed.

In the dental environment, the possible causes of cardiac arrest would include:

- Myocardial infarction in a patient with pre-existing ischaemic heart disease
- Adverse reaction to a drug administered in the dental practice
- Secondary to hypoxia as a result of the side-effects of the administration of a sedative agent

In all cases, an area of increasing emphasis within ALS is the prevention of cardiac arrest. Often, there are warnings of impending cardiac arrest. If the warning signs are recognized and acted upon, then the cardiac may be prevented. As the survival from cardiac arrest is only about 50%, prevention has to be better than cure.

In the dental environment, with the drugs and equipment that are recommended in Chapter 1, any treatment in the dental surgery will be simple. The priority will be early access to the emergency services. Examples of conditions where early access would be appropriate are shown in Table 10.1

Table 10.1 Indications to summon additional medical help

System/process affected	Pathology
Airway	Deteriorating
Breathing	Respiratory rate >30 breaths per minute
	Respiratory rate <6 breaths per minute
Circulation	Pulse rate <40 beats per minute
	Pulse rate >140 beats per minute
Neurology	Prolonged or repeated seizures
	Sudden decrease in level of consciousness
Other	Any patient causing significant concern

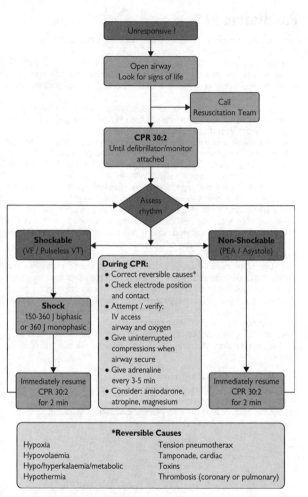

Fig. 10.5 Adult advanced life support algorithm. Reproduced with permission from the Resuscitation Council (UK)

Paediatric ALS

The main differences in adult and paediatric ALS relate to the differences in adults and children as highlighted in Chapter 9.

In children, unlike adults, non-ventricular fibrillation/ventricular tachycardia arrests are more common. Many paediatric cardiac arrests are primarily respiratory in origin. It is thus important to avoid adverse respiratory incidents in children.

If the airway or breathing of a child is compromised, the oxygen reserves are used up much more rapidly than in adults. For this reason, any respiratory problem should be dealt with rapidly.

In the unlikely event that the child suffers a cardiac arrest suitable for defibrillation, the charge delivered is reduced. The protocol for the first three shocks would be 2 joules per kilogram body weight, then a further 2 joules per kilogram body weight, followed by 4 joules per kilogram body weight. Should the cycle have to be repeated, all shocks would be delivered at a charge of 4 joules per kilogram body weight.

The administration of drugs can be different in paediatric patients. Intravenous access can be difficult due to the veins being small and the greater deposits of subcutaneous fat in the younger child. If intravenous access is not possible, drugs can be administered via the intraosseous route. This involves using a special needle to access, just below the knee joint, the bone marrow space of the tibia. The needle punctures the cortical plate of bone and allows fluid to be injected into the cancellous space. The absorption of drugs from this route is so rapid as to be as effective as intravenous administration. The technique is similar in concept to intraosseous local anaesthesia, but the cortical plate can be punctured without the use of a bur in a handpiece!

As with all drug administration, the dose required by an infant or a child is smaller than the adult dose and is based on the child's body weight.

Paediatric ALS algorithm

The philosophy of paediatric ALS is shown in the algorithm in. Fig. 10.6 The Resuscitation Council runs separate training courses for paediatric ALS, as opposed to adult ALS. There is no paediatric equivalent of adult ILS.

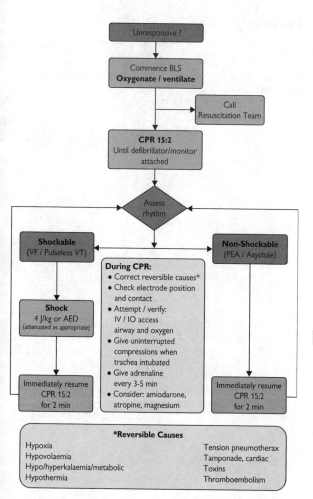

Fig. 10.6 Paediatric advanced life support. Reproduced with permission from the Resuscitation Council (UK)

Summary

Only those members of the dental team involved in treating patients under general anaesthesia or using advanced sedation techniques are required to be competent in ALS or paediatric ALS procedures. Those who initiate the chain of survival should, however, be aware of the events later in the chain.

Index

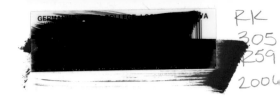

For Reference

Not to be taken from this room

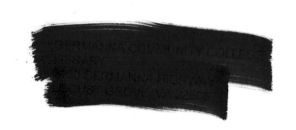